The Question of
Healing Services

The Question of Healing Services

JOHN RICHARDS

daybreak
London

First published in 1989 by
Daybreak
Darton, Longman and Todd Ltd
89 Lillie Road, London SW6 1UD

British Library Cataloguing in Publication Data

Richards, John, *1939–*
  The question of healing services
  1. Christian church. Ministry of healing
  I. Title
  265′.82

ISBN 0–232–51762–2

Phototypeset by Input Typesetting Ltd,
London SW19 8DR
Printed and bound in Great Britain by
Anchor Press Ltd, Tiptree, Essex

Dedicated
in gratitude
to my fellow representatives
on the
Churches' Council for Health and Healing

also
in affectionate memory of
Mother Mary Clare SLG
who has been a source of
'immeasurable riches'
throughout my ministry.

Contents

Author's Note

In order to contain a considerable amount of material within limits, I have not included many quotations, or peppered the text with references and footnotes. To offset this I have appended lists of the authoritative documents (whose teaching I am handing down) and fuller details of the major books and organizations mentioned.

The Church's Healing Ministry has never been far from my thoughts since my crippled mother was instantly healed when anointed over twenty-five years ago.* I have learnt much over that period from the holiness, wisdom, publications – and mistakes! – of others. Please forgive my inability now to excavate and record all the sources of my present thinking, and hence failure to thank those to whom I am indebted. My bibliography begins, however, to do this, as well as providing a guide to further reading.

The *Jerusalem Bible* has been used unless otherwise stated (published and copyright 1966, 1967 and 1968 by Darton, Longman and Todd Ltd and Doubleday & Co. Inc. by permission of the publishers). Since conflicting theories of authorship do not undermine the authority of Scripture, I have – for ease and clarity – bypassed all questions of who wrote what and used the names most obvious to the majority of readers.

John Richards
Renewal Servicing

*A full account is given in *We Believe in Healing*.

1

Understanding

My aims in writing this are:
1. To provide the necessary *background* to understand the wide variety of practices within the Church's Ministry of Healing.
2. To set public healing services in the above *context*.
3. To respond to the many *questions* they raise – whether by those 'for' or 'against'.
4. To relay the balanced and *authoritative teaching* of the churches rather than give an individual opinion.
5. To give detailed guidelines through the basic decisions and necessary *planning*.
6. To give practical and pastoral help to those who are called to *minister* at them.

Public healing services range from the excellent to the dreadful! My purpose is not to promote yet more of them, but to encourage the good and discourage the weak. This book is about *discerning* what is pastorally and theologically right in a given situation, and basing such discernment on sound teaching and clear insight.

The non-medical healing scene is littered with quacks and cults who promote some truth to the exclusion of all else. That is the error of heresy. My slightly cryptic chapter headings are a device to discourage you from focusing just on the part that attracts you and discarding the whole!

I am concerned here with healing services that take place *publicly* rather than in home or hospital (because ample guidance exists for such ministering to the sick).

Problem?

Imagine a small committee gathered to plan a healing service.

Chairman: I've asked Fr Highest from St Isosceles and All Angles to help me with the Laying-on-of-hands . . .

Bill: Just two? It'll take all night!

Betty: Anyway why can't those *not* ordained lay on hands? Our church secretary is a G.P. Why don't you let *her* help you?

George: We need to decide now whether it is to be a Communion Service or not. If it is, there will be some from other denominations whose discipline will not . . .

Fiona: Other denominations! Who said anything about letting anyone else in?! People need to be prepared.

Chairman: Er . . . the Eucharist is *the* healing service . . .

Bill: That's fine, let's scrap the idea altogether!

Ernest (Bible at the ready): Nonsense! What *really* matters is that the Lord is 'present to heal' as we read in Luke 5:17. Sacraments have their place, but Scripture teaches that 'The Lord inhabiteth the praise of his people'. We must have lots of 'prayer n' *praise*'.

Chairman: 'Prayer and Praise' – what a fine description of the Eucharist, is it not?

Nick: What 'ee wants is them silly jingles goin' on n' on n' on . . .

Organist: Never! Only the finest music is good enough for God! . . .

Bill (in a stage whisper): He'll soon be unemployed!

Organist (continuing): . . . I'm not allowing any cheap ditties when I'm in charge!

Youth Leader: 'Ere, come awf it! I thought my Rave n' Rock Revival Group was going to lead the singing. You can't leave us out!

Fiona: Healing's nothing to do with *young* people!

Youth Leader: They've great appeal for the masses!

Fiona: Masses – who wants *them*!! You weren't contemplating letting in outsiders, were you?

Chairman: Well, er . . . yes . . . and . . . er . . . no!

Ernest: 'That the world might believe!' If God is going to do something let's go out into the hedgerows and byways and *compel* them to come in.

Bill: There ain't no 'edgerows near 'ere!

Mary: What about the ill who can't tolerate sitting in one place for more than half-an-hour?

Bill: Get 'em 'ealed in the first thirty minutes then you won't 'ave a problem, will you!

Chairman (coughing gently): Ah, very droll indeed.

Betty: It would save a lot of time if we did what I experienced at a conference. Let the members of the congregation just gather into small natural groups and pray for one another . . .

Chairman: Quick! Smelling salts for Mrs Entwhistle!

Ernest: Let's pray for her . . .

Bill: No, she wants *air* not prayer!

My mild parody demonstrates why this book is entitled '*The Question* of Healing Services'! It serves also to highlight the range of styles and approaches.

Is such variety chaotic? Enriching? or a complex mixture of both?

The Varieties

There is so much variation within the Church's Ministry of Healing that you may wonder whether there is a central core of agreement at all! Take the authors! Are David Watson, Leslie Weatherhead, Anne White, John Wimber, Edward Winckley, John Wilkinson, Jim Wilson, and Michael Wilson all *really* writing about the same thing?

Do they reflect some thinking *in* the Church or the thinking *of* the Church?

What is the mind of the Church on healing?

Is there an overall view that can contain all this variety and make some sense of it?

Emphatically *yes*.

The following chapters contain such an overall view and the mind of the Church. In writing them I have aimed for clarity above all else, believing a black-and-white picture of the whole to be infinitely more useful than a detailed colour picture of a part.

My experience of healing services around the country has demonstrated (among other things) how very easy it is to get things wrong. It is as if a public healing service magnifies and exposes the weaknesses in our thinking and preparation. There is nothing in the healing ministry that demands so much thought, and nothing which so richly rewards it.

I recall one service which ran about two hours over schedule because the arrangers assumed that intensive counselling should be available to all! They probably accomplished their aim, or, more likely, had no specific aims at all!

The all-important overall view of the Church's Ministry of Healing requires us to be aware of (a) the four main *views* of it; (b) its *development* and (c) its three main *streams*.

The Four Main Views

1. The 'Popular' View

The first view of the Church's Healing Ministry is the 'popular' one, based either on 'faith healers' or 'spiritual healers'. Both usually work without reference either to Church or Medicine.

(a) FAITH HEALERS

They generally have well-advertised travelling ministries and promise 'healing' to all who have 'faith' (neither is ever defined!). Faith healers demonstrate 'divine healing' and strive to raise hopes and emotions to accomplish seemingly instant cures. Their style is 'religious', and they claim that their abilities are of God. Physical relief is the goal; medicine and psychiatry are often scorned, and death is a disaster. It later falls to the local clergy and doctors to pastor those whose hopes – and sometimes lives – are shattered.

(b) SPIRITUAL HEALERS

The so-called 'Spiritualist Church' is, in spite of its name, neither of the Spirit nor of the Church! It is responsible for *the majority of advertised public healing services*. Its style is counterfeit Christian, with prayers and hymns (with references to the Atonement expurgated!). Its popularity is due to the

5

failure of the Church to preach an Easter Faith and to teach the reality of the Communion of Saints. The 'Spiritualist' Church offsets these deficiencies by encouraging contact with the dead through mediums (now termed 'sensitives') and heals by evoking and claiming the aid of *spirits*, departed or otherwise. The late Harry Edwards claimed the constant spirit-aid of Pasteur and Lister! (Witchcraft also promises to heal but its style is not counterfeit Christian so it causes less confusion.)

(c) STRENGTH
The strength of this view is its healthy suspicion of fringe healing activities, of spirit-healing, of unauthorized and untrained ministry, and of emotionalism.

(d) WEAKNESS
This lies in its failure to discern that apart from the outward expression of laying-on-hands *such healers' activities are almost the exact opposite of the Church's Ministry of Healing and have nothing to do with it*. This view is, however, widespread and regularly perpetuated in the popular press and magazines. It is a sad case of *mistaken identity* and it is the largest factor in the rejection by Christians of their Church's Healing Ministry. Folk are entitled to reject what it is, but it is just foolish to reject what it *isn't*!

2. The 'Booster' View

This view is the simplest to grasp, and stems from Luther and Calvin. While it accepts the miraculous elements of the New Testament it holds that God withdrew them from the Church, using them not unlike booster rockets to assist the Church in its initial launching. Calvin wrote:

The gift of healing disappeared with the other miraculous powers which the Lord was pleased to give for a time, that it might render the new preaching of the gospel ever more wonderful. Therefore even if we were to grant that anointing was a sacrament of those powers which were then administered by the hands of the apostles, it pertains not to us to whom no such powers have been committed.[1]

The argument that wonders were withdrawn to make preaching 'more wonderful' seems to me a little lame! The Prayer Book reflects this view, and it is held by a distinguished army of saints and scholars of the 'reformed' traditions. There are certainly some Biblical pointers in this direction, which I shall discuss later. The Christian Medical Fellowship in publishing Edmunds and Scorer's *Some Thoughts on Faith Healing* probably endorse their holding this view (p. 62).

(a) STRENGTH
(i) This 'booster' view stems from a desire to affirm the uniqueness of the New Testament, and
(ii) to re-establish the authority of the Word.
(iii) It affirms medicine as God's major means of healing.
(iv) Less positively it enables a non-healing church on the one hand to affirm the authority of Scripture in all matters of faith and conduct, while on the other seemingly to ignore Spiritual teaching and practice regarding the sick.

(b) WEAKNESS
(i) Studies show[2] that the healing ministry did *not* die with the Apostles.

7

(ii) The Eastern Church has never ever held this view.

(iii) For the first thirteen centuries the Western Church never held it either.

(iv) Luther later changed his mind! His friend Melanchthon was 'visibly brought from the point of death' by Luther's prayers.[3] Luther later advised on healing ministry and even wrote a form of healing service based on James 5:13ff.

(v) Both Biblical and modern thought agree on the essential *unity* of the human personality. Anything less than the whole Gospel for the whole person is inadequate. It is as much an error to ignore the body as it is to be preoccupied with it.

3. The 'Recent' View

There has been an explosion of interest and activity in the healing ministry in the last twenty or so years, particularly within the charismatic/renewal movement. This has led many to assume that the Church's Ministry of Healing in the UK is comparatively recent and was heralded by e.g. Francis MacNutt. I shall say more about this charismatic development later. Meanwhile we need to note its strength and weakness.

(a) STRENGTH

(i) It testifies to a world-wide explosion of authentic Christian experience of God's Holy Spirit to renew and heal, in what the Vatican has described as this 'Springtime of the Church'.

(ii) It reflects a massive injection of teaching through publications, tapes, seminars and conferences.

(iii) It arises from the steady increase in the practice of the healing ministry at all local levels.

(b) WEAKNESS
(i) It is strongly influenced by imported teaching.
(ii) This often leads to immaturity and to inheriting the weaknesses of Pentecostalist theology and practice.

4. The 'Modern History' View

This view sees today's healing ministry as the peak of a hundred years' growth. History proves its accuracy. Only from knowing what has been learnt over this longer period can the mind of the Church be known. I shall summarize this in the next chapter.

(a) STRENGTH
(i) It is historically sound.
(ii) If the mind of the Church is sought it is the best starting point.

(b) WEAKNESS
(i) It can assume that to know much is to know all.
(ii) It can rest on the past rather than build on it.

These are not the only views, but they are the main ones relevant to the question of healing services. (Some hold that God does not exist or cannot be encountered, others that he does not or cannot act in history. These views are not unimportant, but I can pass by them here, since those who hold them will not want guidance about holding services of Christian healing!)

We may always learn from the views of others. Each of the four views I have highlighted may serve as a useful reminder.

The 'Popular' view reminds us not to confuse the Church's Ministry of Healing with the much more publicized and popular activities of 'spiritual healers' and 'faith healers'.

The '*Booster*' view prompts us to give due weight to the unique witness and teaching of the New Testament.

The '*New*' view alerts us to discern any new word of the Spirit to the Church to develop or deepen this ministry.

The '*Modern History*' view shows us the vast store of wisdom and experience already given by the Spirit and on which we should draw, if we are to avoid two errors. The first is to be so blinkered that we 'start at square one' when the Holy Spirit is in fact leading the Church from square ten to square eleven!

The second error (which stems from the first) is to assume that the 'latest' is the 'best', and to confuse the part with the whole. When this happens new individual contributions given by God to enrich the Church's Healing Ministry merely fragment it.

I was once invited to address a healing conference for doctors and clergy. I was due to speak in the afternoon, but arrived after morning coffee to get the feel of it. They spent two wearisome hours beginning to grapple with a key topic but made little headway; it defeated them.

Just as the chairman was about to conclude for lunch I ventured a contribution.

'The question you have been considering', I said, 'has been studied and thought through long ago. May I read just two sentences from a report I have here?' They agreed and I did. What a relief! Smiles all round! No longer defeated they went off to enjoy lunch!

Any secular company learns to build on its past experience or folds up. Why not the Church? What a *waste* of time and talent for clergy and doctors to spend a morning grappling with questions that have occupied others for years but which have been already answered in just two sentences! (Many such sentences – from the same report – will appear in the next chapter.)

There are countless burning issues today of which we do not know the answers. We owe it to today's sufferers not to waste time. It can hardly be God's will that we should be travelling on spiritually square wheels unaware of their later important development!

What follows is a whistle-stop tour from 'square one' to 'square ten' looking at lessons learned along the way.

1. Quoted in *Healing and Christianity*. Note: further details of principal titles listed on pp. 170ff.
2. E.g. *Christian Healing, Healing and Christianity* and *Healing Miracles*.
3. From *Healing and Christianity*.

2

Learning

John Gunstone in his recent book *The Lord is Our Healer* gives a useful summary of the healing ministry through the centuries, and traces the roots of this century's revival back through Edward Irving, the Holiness Movements, and John Wesley.

This century's rediscovery is divided into three phases by the two World Wars, for it was over a hundred years ago that a major international conference on 'Divine Healing' was held in London.

Phase One: Missions and Guilds

The 'sacramental' and 'charismatic' streams are nothing new. In 1904, for instance, the Bishop of Salisbury, a great scholar and ecumenist, wrote on the Anglican view of healing for the benefit of Eastern Orthodox Christians. Another famous scholar, Dr Percy Dearmer, an authority on liturgy, ceremonial and church music, founded (with others) the *Guild of Health* to promote a right understanding of the Church's Ministry of Healing and its true relationship to Medicine. Part of its task was to counter the heresies of Christian Science and other healing movements which had arisen to compensate for the Church's deficiency in the matter.

In the same year, 1904, a little removed geographically but *far* removed in style, Evan Roberts, the young son of a miner, had a mighty experience of God which drove him to preach virtually non-stop for six months. Since 1890 he had prayed to be 'Spirit-filled', and his intense ministry of preaching and healing is termed now the 'Welsh Revival'. This movement was one of the foundation streams of the Pentecostalist churches and their healing-evangelists.

At about this time too, an Anglican layman with a gift, or 'charism', of healing founded what is now called the Divine Healing Mission. His name was James Moore Hickson. The then Archbishop of Canterbury was so impressed by Hickson's pamphlet *The Healing Christ in the Church* that he gave copies to the world-wide gathering of bishops at the 1908 Lambeth Conference!

They considered the subject with due care and caution.

It took them *fifty years* to tackle the subject fully and authoritatively, and I will be summarizing their conclusions below.

Mr Hickson, who had received his healing gift at the age of fourteen, was commissioned for world-wide ministry. He toured America, Canada, India, Japan, South Africa, New Zealand and Australia. In each area he received the bishop's backing and filled the cathedrals! The Australian bishops wrote a remarkable document of testimony to the Lord's healing work through him in his services, and in due course he published his own account in *Heal the Sick*.

There were miracles at home too.

Dorothy was dying of tubercular peritonitis. For the previous two weeks she had been deaf, blind and frequently unconscious.

13

Her breathing stopped.

Eight minutes later she sat up and said, 'I am well now!', got up, walked and soon asked for a meal! Her proclamation of Christ's healing power hit the headlines of 1912. Her X-rays showed that new lungs had replaced the ones eaten away with consumption. Like Mr Hickson, Dorothy Kerin was later commissioned for healing missions here and abroad.

The pressure upon the physician to heal *himself* (Luke 4:23) is always present in the Church's Healing Ministry. It seems to me no accident that God raised up a layman and a laywoman for this world-wide work. They were important symbols for the healing of potential rifts between the ordained and the laity, and between male and female leadership.

A 'divided healing-Church' is something of a contradiction in terms. Not surprisingly, therefore, after its first ten years the (Anglican) Guild of Health felt that healing could not be adequately or authentically considered or practised behind the man-made walls of denominationalism. In 1915 the Guild became ecumenical. Non-conformists and Free-churchmen were then less interested than they are today in the sacramental approach, especially anointing, and lest the sacramental insights dwindled the Guild of St Raphael was formed for Anglicans.

The guilds' quarterly magazines, now *Way of Life* and *Chrism* respectively, have thus each served the churches for over seventy years.*

---

* Further details of all organisations mentioned are listed on p. 176. When names over the years have changed I have, for clarity, used today's forms.

Phase Two: Homes and Services

The inter-war years continued things well, although James Moore Hickson's hopes for a healing home were dashed in 1910 by the General Medical Council (GMC) who threatened to strike off the Register any doctor who worked in conjunction with a medically unqualified person. Hickson deserved no such a rebuff. He had deliberately taken courses on anatomy and physiology; welcomed medical co-operation, and saw no patients without their doctors' consent.

In 1928, to his joy, a former patient found, for his own Divine Healing Mission, a residential healing home and headquarters at Crowhurst. (There are now about twenty-five healing centres run by different Christian groups.) His patient was the Revd Howard Cobb, the first of a noble line of Wardens later to include the Revd George Bennett, author of *Miracle at Crowhurst, Heart of Healing*, etc.

A healing service has been the weekly focus at Crowhurst since its foundation, but in 1928 there were scarcely any authorized forms of healing services to be used. The reasons for this arose much earlier.

Although to 'reform' means essentially to 'improve', as far as the Church's Ministry of Healing was concerned the Reformers did no such thing. By their over-reaction to abuse they deprived Christians of much of God's healing grace for two-and-a-half centuries. At the time the Roman Catholic Church had slipped into anointing only the dying as a preparation for death ('Extreme Unction').

The Reformers made the gross mistake of trying to solve the problem of *mis*-use by *non*-use rather

15

than *right* use. So their Prayer Book replaced the Service of Extreme Unction by a Service for the Visitation of the Sick – a service of 'extreme melancholy'! The so-called 'Reformers' did not reform anointing but abolished it. The Roman Catholics, by contrast, in their Counter Reformation did what the Reformers failed to do and made their practice of anointing more Biblical!

The Book of Common Prayer, although Anglican, profoundly influenced all the reformed churches, so its view of sickness became the norm. Its service encouraged the view that sickness is a punishment for sin (still widely held!). It urged the patient to make his will and settle his debts – for 'the quietness of his executors'! It denied the patient both Anointing and the Laying-on-of-hands. I imagine the only ones to regard this development as an improvement were the undertakers!

(Even the Great Awakening of the nineteenth century was unable to right things, and, except in Pentecostalism, most evangelism in the Western Church still has little healing content either for the individual or society.)

Clergy had anointed the sick in the London Diocese since before 1900, so after the Great War there was considerable pressure to include Anointing and the Laying-on-of-hands in the proposed Revised Prayer Book of 1928. Although Parliament rejected the revised book, its influence was considerable and the Laying-on-of-hands was restored.

Spiritualism was rejected by the Lambeth Conference of 1920, along with Christian Science. The latter is neither Christian nor Scientific! It rejects major Biblical doctrines and alleges that only mind is real and that matter has no reality. Pain and disease are an illusion caused by wrong thinking.

16

Christian Scientists hold services with Scripture readings, hymns and they administer 'spiritual healing'. For most people the vivid experience of sitting on a pin is sufficient to disprove such heresy!

After a decade's work the Anglican bishops worldwide fully affirmed the Church's Ministry of Healing. They:

(i) Urged the recognition of spiritual gifts.

(ii) Encouraged clergy-doctor co-operation.

(iii) Regarded all disease as an evil to be combatted.

(iv) Saw healing in terms of the 'whole person'.

(v) Recommended the formation of prayer groups.

(vi) Encouraged ministry through prayer, and through the 'sacramental' acts of Laying-on-of-hands and Anointing. (Christians vary a little in what they call a 'sacrament' and in which ones they believe to have been instituted by Christ himself. It is usually taken to mean an outward sign of something spiritual, e.g. the Breaking of Bread. The Salvation Army reject sacraments, but their understanding of a warm Christian greeting would, I am sure, be 'sacramental'.)

Anointing was understood as it was earlier in both the East and West to be for the *healing of the whole person*.

Further encouragement was given with the publication of 'authorized' forms of service for such ministry. Although provision was made for their taking place privately, the assumption was that when possible Anointing or Laying-on-of-hands would take place *within the public worship of the Eucharist*, i.e. public services with healing, if not exactly public healing services. They form the basis of virtually all such liturgy today.

In contrast the bishops were *un*willing to give any 'encouragement to Public Healing Missions'. Earlier they had authorized and supported the world-wide 'public healing missions' of James Moore Hickson and Dorothy Kerin. Was this a U-turn? I think not. It recognized that such folk were the exceptions to prove the rule, and that most public healing mission ministries were led by Spiritualists or faith healers.

A distinction might usefully be made between evangelistic missions of which healing is a *by-product*, those designed to *demonstrate* healing, and those which aim to *teach* it. Where there is adequate teaching, the problem of the lack of preparation is largely overcome.

Phase Three: Expansion and Definition

There is a directory published by the Churches' Council for Health and Healing (CCHH) which lists about *fifty* entries directly related to the Church's Ministry of Healing. It is beyond the scope of this publication even to list them, let alone relate their history! Here is just a random sample – The Guild of Health; The Guild of St Raphael; The Guild of Pastoral Psychology; The Order of St Luke; The Baptist Union Health and Healing Group; The Healing and Pastoral Committee of the Methodist Church; The United Reformed Church Ministry of Healing Committee; The Friends' Fellowship of Healing; The Christian Fellowship of Healing (Scotland); The Church's Ministry of Healing (Ireland); The Institute of Religion and Medicine; The Hospital Chaplaincy Council; The Clinical Theology Association; The Dorothy Kerin Trust; Caring Professions Concern; Wholeness Through Christ; The Other Ministry of Health; The St Marylebone Centre; The Acorn Trust; Green Pastures Home of

Healing, etc. and etc! (If you would like the complete list they are included in *Your Very Good Health*, further details on p. 173.)

If you skipped that last paragraph I am not worried, its very size makes my point! My purpose is not to teach you history but to open your eyes to the real situation. (Readers who *are* interested in the history I would refer to Bishop Maddocks' *The Christian Healing Ministry*.)

I shall not relate the post-War developments, but confine my comments to just two key items – one council and one publication.

The Council

What is now the Churches' Council for Health and Healing was initiated in 1944. In its present form it consists of over eighty representatives. These come from three areas – the churches and denominations, the healing homes, and the royal medical colleges and related disciplines. Its influence and work are authoritative and considerable.

Its offices, together with the offices of many other healing guilds, are at St Marylebone Parish Church, London. Space precludes my telling the story of how an Anglican Church in the Harley Street area now has an NHS practice in its crypt – as part of a bold step towards offering full healing for the whole person.

The Publication

I have mentioned that it took the Lambeth Conference fifty years to reach their conclusions about the

Church's Ministry of Healing. In 1958 their balanced – and certainly not hasty! – assessment was distilled in a commission report entitled *The Church's Ministry of Healing*.

This encapsulated the Church's thinking on the matter as it had developed and deepened over half a century. It asks – and answers – ninety-five per cent of the questions that are usually raised concerning healing. Although Anglican, virtually all other denominations have since taken the same line. It is, without doubt, the most authoritative document to date.

Unfortunately, during the last twenty years – when it was needed most – it was out of print! My recent abridgement of it has been published and makes it available again under the slightly different title *The Church's Healing Ministry*.* Lord Coggan in his foreword writes, 'The Report contains a great deal of wisdom which is still needed today. It would be a considerable loss to the Church if we were deprived of this just because the Report has gone out of print.' There is no comparable document that expresses the mind of the Church on its healing ministry. Many of its conclusions have considerable practical repercussions in any thinking and planning about healing services.

One of the Report's most useful features is to expose common misconceptions. (The references to 'CHM §49, §126' etc. are to the numbered paragraphs in my current abridged edition.)

* Published by Marshall Pickering and Renewal Servicing.

Misconceptions

(i) The Faith Misconception

This is *that healing inevitably follows faith* (CHM §57–61). The assumption that the sick may expect 'healing' if their 'faith' is strong enough, and the corresponding deduction that unhealed sickness indicates a lack of faith is contrary both to Scripture and experience. It is cruel to those who remain sick. This teaching is widespread and increasing. Detailed arguments against it are in my pamphlet *Faith & Healing*, while below (pp. 65–7) I have analysed the Biblical material.

(ii) The Suffering Misconception

This is *that suffering is always contrary to God's will* (CHM §62–3). Pain is essentially a warning system. Although disease is always to be fought, Gethsemane and the Cross demonstrate against this misconception. Some suffering may have a redemptive or other positive purpose. Most healing takes place gradually and continued suffering does not preclude healing. Sometimes, as my dental visits remind me, suffering seems to be necessary for healing!

(iii) The Healing Misconception

Following from the last is the wrong belief that *God must heal* (CHM §64), by which is usually meant instant and physical cure. This view of healing is altogether too narrow.

(iv) The Death Misconception

This arises from these earlier misconceptions, i.e. if suffering is always contrary to God's will and he must heal, then *death is always a disaster*. This denies our Easter Faith. Since our view of life depends largely upon our view of death it is an inadequate life-view for the Christian (CHM §65–6).

(v) The Sin Misconception

This assumes that *sin is the cause of all sickness*. Jesus repudiated this (John 9:3). Although there is often a relationship – particularly with corporate sin, wars, etc. – it is not generally true of the individual. If sickness were God's just punishment for sin Jesus would not have removed it – or, if he had, his Father would have told him to put it back again! The gospel brings hope not despair. God is not a God of revenge, although this belief surfaces strongly whenever there is what we interestingly term 'un-deserved suffering'.

(vi) The Medicine Misconception

This assumes *that modern medicine has superseded the Church's Ministry of Healing* (CHM §70–7). Put simply: medicine can make people better, but cannot make them *whole*. While an individual Christian doctor may bestow peace, forgiveness, acceptance of Christ, or faith in God, it is not within the competence of medicine as such to do so. These deeper needs remain, and the Church has a mission to all mankind to teach, preach and heal (Matt. 4:23, 9:35).

(vii) The Healer Misconception

This misconception is *that the Church's Ministry of Healing lies in the hands of the specially gifted* (CHM §78–82). Witches can cure. Invisible healing powers may not be Christian, but occult or even demonic. The ministry belongs at the centre. Ministers should not hold back because of an apparent lack of healing gifts for Christ's authority has been entrusted to them.

(viii) The Fringe Misconception

This is *that the Church's Ministry of Healing is separate from its other work*. The Report insists that the importance of this ministry 'must not lead to setting it apart in any way' (CHM §83–4).

(ix) The Physical Misconception

It is commonly held that *physical healing is all that matters*. It does matter greatly, of course, but full physical abilities are to Christians neither the goal of life nor the guarantee of happiness. There are many very fit people who suffer profound 'dis-ease', and many handicapped whose 'wholeness/holiness' is an inspiration (CHM §85–6).

(x) Other Misconceptions

The Report mentions others. (a) That sacramental ministries herald death. (b) That a medically unexplained healing is more wonderful than a medically explained one. (c) That it is a fallacy to assume that events preceding a change are automatically its cause.

The relevance of these to the planning of public

healing services will be obvious and cannot be over-estimated. When these misconceptions are avoided then the hallmark of the true Christian ministry begins to emerge. The prevalence of the nine basic *mis*conceptions may suggest to you that healing services ought *not* to be introduced without teaching!

Terminology

The Report rejects three popular terms because they are so misleading. There is important teaching here:

(i) 'Faith Healing'

This was rejected (CHM §21) because of the dangerous misconceptions associated with it. Non-Christian healers rarely define either 'faith' or 'healing'. The 'faith' need have no religious content whatsoever, but may rest in e.g. the healer's abilities.

(ii) 'Spiritual Healing'

Although rightly used this refers to the work of the Holy Spirit, it is used by the so-called Spiritualist Church which ministers through the alleged powers of departed or other spirits. There is enough confusion without the Church calling its ministry 'spiritual healing' (CHM §22)!

(iii) 'Divine Healing'

This too is rejected by the 1958 Commission (but nobly retained by e.g. The Divine Healing Mission founded over fifty years earlier). The anxiety behind this phrase was the implication that only when the

Christian *Church* ministers is it 'divine', and that God was in no way in the work of medicine. Medicine is based on the Laws of Nature which Christians see as the Laws of God. There is a right sense in which the Creator is at work in medicine – see below pp. 59–63 (CHM §23).

(iv) The Chosen Term

The reason for rejecting these popular terms is to avoid confusion and misunderstanding, and to safeguard the Christian ministry. The term adopted and used for the last thirty years is '*The Church's Ministry of Healing*'. (It is a bit of a give-away if you do not use it!)

It avoids ambiguity. It rejects any link with faith-healers and Spiritualism. It fosters its relationship to medicine. It affirms that this ministry belongs not to Christian individuals – however saintly or gifted – but to the *Church*.

When we apply the mind of the Church to healing services such things make a quite practical difference.

For instance, if I am asked to preach at a healing service it is invariably assumed that I will also assist with the Laying-on-of-hands. I resist this. There are many famous 'names' who accept such invitations and hog the show! This inevitably strengthens the misconception that this ministry belongs to certain individuals rather than the local church.

Beliefs and practice cannot be separated. Wrong beliefs lead to wrong practices. It is no good holding right beliefs about the healing ministry and then so thoughtlessly arranging things that they reinforce such misconceptions!

If it really *is* the *Church's* Healing Ministry then

what we do in its name should reinforce this. My own practice of *not* engaging both in the ministry of preaching and the ministry of the Laying-on-of-hands has often been commented on with great surprise yet deep approval by members of congregations. If I have prepared and given a major preaching ministry I am pretty exhausted, and later in the service sometimes naturally join with others to receive God's individual blessing to renew, refresh and re-equip me.

Although I do this quite naturally and not in any way whatever to demonstrate anything, I have often been told that to see me *receiving* ministry does speak powerfully against the all-too-common assumptions that God's power and presence are specially imported for the occasion and are exclusively focused in the person of some itinerant spiritual whizz-kid!

The truth that 'The Lord is here! His Spirit is with us!' depends not on the abilities and punctuality of British Rail to deliver visiting speakers, but on God's own promise and faithfulness. Where such occasions are well prepared the appearance or otherwise of some outside speaker will make little or no difference to the service being a truly healing one!

3

Seeing

There are *three streams* of healing in the British churches. Their age is directly related to their size – the oldest is by far the largest, and the most recent is the smallest. The dates 1900, 1960 and 1984 indicate roughly the start of each.

Virtually every service, publication, style of ministry, terminology, and type of teaching are directly related to one or other of these three streams. Failure to discern this renders the scene a bewildering hotchpotch of apparent contradictions – some of which I illustrated in my fictional planning committee at the beginning of chapter one!

Once these 'streams' are understood, then the seeming contradictions, varieties of ministry, plethora of styles and contrasts in teaching and terminology begin to form some sort of rich unity.

In some of my earlier writings I taught that there were only two streams, for such was then the case, and I labelled the first stream 'sacramental'. The ministry of John Wimber has in recent years created a third stream, which is likely to swell. I have revised also my naming the first stream 'sacramental'. It accurately captures its ethos, but might be misleading if it was taken to imply that the other streams were *non*-sacramental. I have renamed the first stream –

The Mature Stream

The previous chapter outlined much of its development and some of its teaching. It is in this octogenarian tradition that much of the 'mind of the Church' will be found – but not all. It deserves the flattering label I have given it, and for clarity's sake may be analysed as follows –

Strengths

(i) An adequate theology of healing.
(ii) A theology of suffering.
(iii) A theology of dying.
(iv) A sacramental basis.
(v) A strong order and discipline in healing ministry.
(vi) Due place is given to authority.
(vii) Willingness to be guided by past experience.
(viii) A strong confidentiality.
(ix) A loyal affirmation of medicine.
(x) A readiness to learn and work in an interdisciplinary way.

    Maturity is very desirable but it is not everything. Tom Smail once said, '*It is difficult to be mature and aflame at the same time*!' Although I wholeheartedly commend the riches of this tradition I know it well enough not to be blind to its potential weaknesses.

Weaknesses

(i) A tendency not to recognize or use lay gifts.
(ii) A professional caution which fears anything unpredictable.
(iii) A failure to work out the corporate nature of this ministry.
(iv) An in-group view of healing that tends to restrict healing ministry to well-informed churchgoers.

(v) A low-key style that hides this ministry from society.

(vi) Little or no link with mission or evangelism.

(vii) Some lack of expectancy in praying and ministering.

(viii) A tendency to 'shelter' somewhat behind God's sovereign work in the sacraments.

(ix) A failure to develop the right and necessary styles and contexts for sharing.

(x) A widespread failure to relate and develop the immense healing potential of formal confession.

(xi) A tendency to assume the omnicompetence of psychiatry.

(xii) Some slowness in learning new things outside its own 'stream'.

The Charismatic Stream

Although this is often called a 'movement', it follows no individual. It is a phenomenon of spontaneous spiritual combustion! The leadership of various churches has varied in its willingness to understand and readiness to accept it. Among the wisest leadership has been the Roman Catholic. This is due, I suspect, to their greater sense of history, and the realization that there is nothing in charismatic renewal that the Church has not experienced and accepted before. There are now about fifty-million Roman Catholics who would identify with this label.

Anglican bishops regularly pray for those they confirm that they would *daily increase in the Holy Spirit more and more . . .*'. It might, therefore, have been assumed that they had a clearer grasp than most of the Holy Spirit and his workings. If they did, they did not reveal it. The impression given is

29

that most thought that if they shut their eyes for long enough the charismatic phenomenon would go away!

It did not!

The unwillingness of church leaders in general to parent this unplanned spiritual child created problems. There were questions that simply *had* to be answered and if the official leadership of the churches would not provide them, answers would be sought elsewhere.

'What is happening?'

'What does it mean?'

'What should we be doing?'

The Fountain Trust was formed as the need for a foster-parent increased, and it managed – with considerable success – to guide this child through adolescence. It did much to harness the wind and utilize the fire, and by its balanced teaching tried to ensure that the authentic charismatic blessings enriched the Church rather than split it.

Its influence was considerable but limited. A great deal of American teaching via publications, tapes and visiting speakers flooded the gaps unfilled by the Fountain Trust.

When the ecclesiastical ostriches dared to look about them, they had a shock! Their abandoned spiritual child had not died of neglect, but was now a big bouncing adolescent with some disconcerting traits!

If I may continue the analogy, the adolescent was generally relieved and pleased to relate to its real parents again. The leaders, however, covered their embarrassment by hastily producing reports to reassure themselves and others that the parent-child relationship had always been good; there was no question whatever of parental neglect, but that, as we all know, it is of the nature of adolescents to be a bit troublesome!

(I had, at one time, to give a paper to the Working Party of the Anglican Synod on the history of the charismatic movement in the Church of England, for *their* report. My comments above are based on more than hearsay.)

I would analyse the charismatic stream in this way:

Weaknesses

(i) Too little theology of healing.
(ii) Too little theology of suffering.
(iii) Too little theology of dying.
(iv) An over-emphasis on feeling and experience.
(v) It is prone to individualism.
(vi) It holds imbalanced views of authority, treating it either too lightly (in the mainstream churches) or imposing it too heavily (in some 'house' churches).
(vii) A preoccupation with the present experience with little or no reflection upon the past.
(viii) An eagerness to testify which is weak on confidentiality.
(ix) Sometimes God's work in medicine is unrecognized.
(x) An unwillingness to face the nitty-gritty of inter-disciplinary work and study.

The careful reader will have realized that these weaknesses *correspond exactly to the strengths of the earlier 'mature' stream*.

There is a dovetailing of the *most remarkable* kind, for in addition to the *weaknesses* of the charismatic stream being offset by the *strengths* of the 'mature' and older stream, the *strengths* of the renewal stream neatly correspond to the *weaknesses* of the 'mature' stream.

Surely God's hand must be seen in this.

Unfortunately almost all Christian groups are over-concerned about their own identity and tend not to be open, to develop, or actively to complement others.

As I reflect on the complementary nature of the mature and charismatic streams, I am tempted to apply the imagery of Ezekiel's vision of the valley of dry bones.

The mature stream is not unlike the 'bones', and the charismatic stream not unlike the 'breath'. The lesson is that *bones need breath and breath needs bones*. Bones without breath are dead; breath without bones is just hot air! Maturity can so easily lose its flame, and that which is aflame can consider itself fully grown merely because it is fully active.

Strengths

(i) A readiness to recognize lay abilities and gifts.

(ii) An openness to be Spirit-led into new areas and styles.

(iii) Some willingness to explore the corporate nature of healing and its costly outworking through experiments in community living, extended families, and so on.

(iv) A more open view, rather than in-group view of healing.

(v) A willingness not to be dominated by caution.

(vi) Some movement towards integrating healing with mission.

(vii) A real expectancy in praying and ministering.

(viii) Little tendency to 'shelter' behind the sacraments.

(ix) Useful developments in right sharing both for the troubled and also for those in leadership.

(x) A very significant enlargement of the healing of confession into healing-of-the-memories, inner healing, and deliverance.

(xi) An unwillingness to minimize the Church's authentic ministries of healing in deference to psychiatry.

These strengths offset the weaknesses of the mature stream listed earlier.

Obviously I may have 'cooked the books' falsely to dovetail these two streams, but I have no motive to do that. I was myself regularly surprised as, over the years, my experience increasingly confirmed this. If my analysis is, for the main part, accurate, then *God has raised up the healing ministry in the charismatic/renewal stream to complete his work begun in the mature stream.*

If this is so, the repercussions are considerable.

It means that both traditions are incomplete. The difference of the 'other' stream from our own does not indicate that it is 'wrong', but that it is complementary. The other cannot be ignored, for it is God's gift for the correction and enrichment of our own distortions and poverty.

In highlighting the two streams' distinctive characteristics I have had to put asunder what should be joined together. My black-and-white treatment is useful for clarity, but does justice to neither stream.

At best, where the maturity is aflame and the fire is mature a new deeper river is created, and the earlier names of the contributory streams irrelevant. When this happens order and freedom, charism and sacrament, leaders and laity, doctrine and experience each enrich and balance the other.

Such rich diversity in turn reflects our God who is both transcendent yet immanent, just yet merciful, powerful yet vulnerable, dependable yet unpredictable.

The Stream of Revived Pentecostalism

Countless churches have experienced new spiritual life and a healing ministry of new dimensions through the ministry and publications of John Wimber, a humble American.

His books *Power Evangelism* and *Power Healing* are best sellers in spite of the unease felt this side of the Atlantic about 'power' in both these contexts. It was John and his colleagues who flew voluntarily from the States to minister to David Watson.

John Wimber's message is good and timely: our gospel is altogether too verbal. Jesus replied to the Baptist's question by pointing to what could be both *seen and heard* (Luke 7:22). Luke describes his Gospel as an account of what Jesus began *to do and to teach* (Acts 1:1). God's Kingdom comes in both words and works, and the gospel has no no-go areas. It should touch the whole person.

In the Acts of the Apostles there is a happy interplay of words and works, but no fixed relationship between the two. 'Wonders' are never used to capture an audience. The healing of the cripple created a crowd to whom Peter preached (3:12ff), but later it was the increase of the believers that prompted the locals to bring their sick for healing (5:14–15).

Although John Wimber's personal ministry is very much broader, his British hosts have insisted that he speak on 'signs and wonders', and it is this theme for which he is here most known.

Much that comes from the States to our churches lacks any real history or development, and John Wimber's very real contribution is no exception.

As so often there is an important distinction to be made between the movement and the man. I shall

use the term 'Wimberism' not in any derogatory
sense but to make this important distinction.
Followers rarely reach the heights of those who
inspire them.

Many are convinced that John Wimber's insights
are leading the healing ministry forward into new
and exciting paths. Is this third stream yet another
complementary gift of God to enrich yet more what
already exists?

My analysis of the pattern and development of the
first two streams and their interdependence almost
presupposes that this most recent stream will repeat
the process.

One cannot cast doubt on the extent of God's
blessing through it, nor its potency to revive and
power to transform. It is early to judge and time
alone will tell whether it will ultimately enrich the
Church as well as individuals.

I have termed it *Revived Pentecostalism* to indicate
that it is basically a revival of something old not an
arrival of something new.

It bears a striking resemblance to the Holiness and
Pentecostalist movements out of which our present
healing ministry grew sixty or seventy years ago. If
so, then we have come full circle and, in British
terms, this is not a glimpse of the future, but 'where
we came in'.

The contribution of the Pentecostalists and their
retaining of what the mainstream churches had lost
place the latter ever in their debt. On their foundations this century's healing ministry was built. This
does not mean to say that they held every truth in
perfect balance. Over the years their strengths were
assimilated and their weaknesses discerned.

In their early years the Pentecostalists considered
it sinful to take medicine or go to a doctor if you

had received Christian ministry for healing. Some pastors faced charges of manslaughter for not allowing their dying children medical aid. In 1920 the Pentecostal Holiness Church split over the issue.

With this intolerance of medicine went the tendency to have an upgraded demonology, and mentally to 'locate' God in the supernatural.

As the Church matured in its thinking, it modified each of these. Medicine was affirmed as an area of God's working rather than rejected. The inflated demonology was reduced to size to leave greater room for sin and individual responsibility. The tendency to 'locate' God exclusively in the supernatural was modified to affirm him in the natural as well.

In John Wimber's teaching these themes occur but not always at their most mature – for America has not had the rich and long development of healing that Britain has experienced.

Howard Booth, a gracious and sympathetic reviewer of John Wimber's *Power Healing* had to note that there is 'no affirmation of medicine as an instrument that God has provided.'[1] John Wimber's use of the term 'divine healing' suggests he does not share the British misgivings about its apparent exclusion of medicine.

As far as demonology is concerned some readers will recall that it was one of John Wimber's team who claimed that Satan had killed David Watson. The assumption that Satan is so powerful as to render the world-wide prayers of the Church and God himself impotent is both unScriptural and unacceptable.

While John Wimber would rightly see God at work in the supernatural, I fear that 'Wimberism' might tend mentally to 'locate' him there. While signs should indeed follow those who believe (Mark

16:16–18) human nature is such that believers all too readily tend to follow the signs!

There is a great spiritual danger here. The more God is met in special experiences, the easier it is mentally to 'locate' him outside of the ordinary. When this happens our spiritual life is kept alive by 'signs and wonders' and is shaken when we are deprived of them.

To seek God only in the supernatural is to deny the message of Christmas and Cross. It removes all hope and comfort from the unhealed sick because they are led to believe that God has forsaken them, rather than is suffering with them. It is the pagans who locate God exclusively in wonders, for Christians he is, if I may coin a phrase, *ordinarily in the ordinary*, i.e. where we need him most!

In a society hooked on materialism, supernatural*ism* is attractive. Sadly it is nothing but the opposite heresy! For if materialism is wrongly world-orientated to the exclusion of God's heaven; supernaturalism is wrongly heaven-orientated to the exclusion of God's world.

I am not equating 'Wimberism' with supernaturalism, but I must confess to a real fear that history may show (what as yet we cannot perceive) that Wimber's revived Pentecostalism is no step forward but many steps back, and that while apparently bringing God nearer in fact pushes him away into the supernatural. I speak with no authority on this, this is only my personal impression and I sincerely hope to be proved wrong.

I regard John Wimber himself as a great man of God and pray that the British churches will have the wisdom to integrate his teaching in a way that furthers the healing ministry rather than sets it back.

While it seems to have the weaknesses of early

Pentecostalism this stream may provide the impetus to bring together, especially in mission, the words and works of the Kingdom. In this area we have much to learn and John Wimber much to contribute.

1. In *Healing is Wholeness*, p. 136.

4

Obeying

Public healing services are sometimes justified on the grounds that 'Jesus never turned away any who came to him in need.' Although this *feels* right to those of us familiar with the healing ministry it is not conclusive.

If Jesus did turn anyone away it would not have been useful material for the Gospel-writers and it would not have been recorded. Not turning away is not the same as inviting.

We all tend to read Scripture in the light of our experience and convictions, and we cannot move forward in our understanding of the Church's Healing Ministry without noting carefully the *full* Scriptural witness.

I bought myself a copy of Donald Guthrie's massive *New Testament Theology* to learn what he had to say about the New Testament theology of healing. I opened the thousand-page tome eagerly, and turned to his two-thousand topic index first with admiration then with disbelief! There was no single reference either to healing or anointing!

It is, however, as much a distortion to maximize the Biblical material as it is to minimize it! It is easy to see too much.

Against the Church's Mandate to Heal

The following points need to be noted by all who assume Scriptural authority to heal. (I shall reflect on each later.)

1. Christ's Commission

Jesus of Nazareth's commissioning of the Twelve need not automatically be the Risen Lord's commissioning of the universal Church. If it is, then there is an emphasis on exorcism and Matthew's disconcerting command to raise the dead – which is literal and should not be spiritualized (10:8, see also 11:5).

2. The Seventy

Since Jesus rejoiced in the completion of their mission, their commission (Luke 10:18) was just a once-off rather than once-and-for-all-time.

3. The Signs

The signs that should follow believers (according to the late appendix to Mark, 16:16–18) consist of five items: exorcism; tongues-speaking; picking up snakes unharmed; protection from accidental poisoning; and healing the sick with the Laying-on-of-hands. If this is authoritative (and its late date may reflect established church practice) then why are three promoted but two ignored in the Church's ministry today? Healing the sick comes last! Is not the poison promise relevant to drinking from the same cup as an AIDS sufferer?

4. Epistles

If healing is an integral part of the Church's ministry and mission, why is there so little reference in the epistles?

The Gospels and Acts between them give us twenty-two incidents of individual healing (17+5), seven occasions of exorcisms (6+1), and five accounts of raising the dead (3+2). Using the term 'healing' widely this totals thirty-four healings in all.

By contrast in the epistles there are *no* accounts of any individual healings, exorcisms or raisings.

5. Healing Gifts

These are mentioned only in one chapter of the early Corinthian correspondence (1 Cor. 12:9,28,30), and nowhere else in the New Testament. Neither Christ, the Twelve, the Seventy, Peter, Paul or Ananias are said to have them.

6. Anointing the Sick

The passage in James 5:13ff is the only passage in the epistles about the healing ministry. In it, church members who are sick are urged to summon the elders of the church to pray for them and anoint them in the Name of the Lord. The gift of healing is not mentioned.

7. The Unhealed

Not all were healed. Mention is made of Paul's 'thorn-in-the-flesh' (2 Cor. 12:7ff), and it was Epaphroditus's near-fatal illness to which we owe the Epistle to the Philippians (Phil. 2:25–30). In addition Timothy frequently suffered from what most of us would know as 'Mediterranean Tummy' (1 Tim. 5:23), and Trophimus was left sick at Malta (2 Tim. 4:20) – the very place where Paul and Luke healed the sick (Acts 28:9).

We cannot claim a Biblical foundation for healing ministry and ignore these points.

Readers who wish to study all the relevant material are advised to beg, borrow or buy (it is so good I nearly added 'steal'!) Dr John Wilkinson's definitive *Health and Healing: Studies in N.T. Principles and Practice*. As an example of his thoroughness I will mention that Paul's 'thorn' is afforded no less than thirty pages and fifty footnotes! (Further details of this, and all publications mentioned in the text are in the Bibliography.)

A Response to the Case Against

1. Christ's Commission

I will take the commissioning of the Twelve in conjunction with –

2. The Seventy

The witness of Acts is that the Church *assumed its healing ministry*.

There are two accounts of Peter healing individuals (3:1–10, 9:32–5), one of his raising the dead (9:36–41), one account of him ministering to a group (5:15–16) and he was included among those ministering 'wonders and signs' on two occasions in Jerusalem (2:43, 5:12). He did not act as if the commissions were restrictive.

Those who were not of the Twelve or of the

Seventy followed Peter's example and were not restrained by the Church. Acts records Paul ministering two healings; one exorcism; one raising of the dead; two ministries to groups of sick; and ministering with Barnabas 'signs and wonders' at Iconium (14:8–11, 28:8, 16:16–18, 20:9–12, 19:11–12, 28:9, 14:3). He would not have been able to minister at all had his sight not been restored through the ministry of Ananias (9:17–19, 22:12–16) who was neither an Apostle, nor of the Twelve nor of the Seventy, but a layman.

The recorded commissionings may themselves not be universal, but a universal commissioning was assumed by all, including those to whom they had not been given.

3. The Signs

The Church down the ages has not given equal weight to each of these. The snake-handling sects are regarded by all as fringe – or beyond it! If we rearrange the order according to their relevance to our loving God and our neighbour, they emerge as follows – tongues; healing; exorcism; picking-up snakes; protection from accidental poisoning. Tongues relates usually to our love of God; while healing and exorcism express our love of others. The last two (snakes and poison) seem more related to our own preservation. Paul was protected from snake-bite at Malta (Acts 28:3). There is no Scriptural equivalent for drinking poisons unharmed, but the chalice-and-serpent symbol used of St John refers back to what I found to be a very sober, spiritual and moving account in *The Acts of John* of his God being publicly put to the test on John's ability to drink poison unharmed.[1]

43

Contemporary Christian experience does not lack stories of miraculous protection although in our culture snakes and poison do not feature highly!

The critics are right in saying that equal weight is not placed on all the 'signs' mentioned in Mark's longer ending. The lesser importance attached to snakes and poisons seems reasonable enough, and acceptable against the command to love God and neighbour.

4. The Epistles

Paul, the direct or indirect author of many of the epistles that do not mention healing, has had his own healing ministry outlined in section 2 (above). The silence of the Pauline epistles on healing cannot be taken to imply that their author was against healing or wanted to discourage it!

(Although opinions differ greatly about the authorship of each epistle it is worth noting that according to the Acts, Peter, James, John ('Apostles'), Paul, Philip, Barnabas, Stephen and Ananias were all accredited with healings, signs or wonders.)

It is not so very strange that the epistles hardly mention healing. The Eucharist is only dealt with in response to a pastoral problem. The epistles were neither complete handbooks nor historical narratives of events.

5. Gift of Healing

Paul's term is actually a double plural – *gifts of healings*, and thus suggests a whole range of abilities. That no one is described as possessing it when they are exercising it need not surprise us! The writers probably assumed that if they recorded fine teaching or the working of miracles that those concerned had gifts in those directions. No one described Jesus as having a 'gift of teaching'.

6. Anointing

The teaching of James may either reflect church practice of AD 60 or AD 100 (scholars differ). In either case it is not some late development.

When Christ himself sent out the Twelve and commanded them to heal, the earliest account (Mark 6:7–13) records that their way of ministering to the sick was to *anoint them with oil*. James's teaching is not, therefore, a late development. Anointing the sick is in direct succession to early Apostolic ministry and practice. (The reason why Christ himself did not anoint will emerge in chapter 7.)

7. The Unhealed

The mention of four who remained sick in the epistles does not invalidate the healing ministry. It is never assumed that God's healing through the Church will end all suffering any more than God's healing through Medicine. Not all are healed through medicine – it does not invalidate it. The harsh realism of Paul's 'thorn-in-the-flesh' and his suffering adds weight to the authenticity of miraculous events when they are recorded. Apocryphal writings are rejected as untrustworthy because of their unreality. The New Testament's refusal to gloss over suffering and to record the pain and paradoxes of the healed and the unhealed makes its witness to healing that much more reliable.

Such then is a brief response to seven Biblical points that appear not to support the healing ministry. A number of the issues raised will be dealt with more fully later.

Charismatic v. Sacramental?

It is often assumed, because of the impression given by the epistles, that the healing ministry *declined* in New Testament times. In addition, on the slender basis of the early Corinthian reference to 'gifts' and the later James reference to 'elders', it is often presumed that there was a *shift* in New Testament times from healing being exercised by gifted individuals to being placed in the hands of authorized leaders.

There may be some truth in this, but it must not be assumed that every local congregation around the Eastern Mediterranean was uniform, or that Corinth was typical of them all. If, as is my impression, the Corinthian church was a bit way-out, then the majority of churches might well have always used the pattern of James since Jesus's earthly ministry.

Those who teach that there was something of a switch from the 'charismatic' to the 'sacramental' ministries rarely give reasons for the change.

In the light of what I have said above about the dangers of 'supernaturalism' there is a much ignored theme in the New Testament that has great bearing upon the use of healing gifts.

Wonder-working

The working of wonders was nothing new to Christ. The Old Testament recounted the contest between Moses and Pharoah's magicians, and God's People were warned (Deut. 13:1ff) that if a prophet worked miracles and signs *and* his predictions came true he was not thereby a true prophet if he did not draw people to God. (Countless folk today have not learned this and suffered spiritual shipwreck by voluntary submission to the most trivial paranormal event simply because it contained some truth.)

Christ himself encountered non-Christian wonder-workers, and he exposed the counterfeit thus:

> It is not those who say to me, 'Lord, Lord', who will enter the kingdom of heaven but the person who does the will of my Father in heaven . . . many will say to me, 'Lord, Lord, did we not prophesy in your name, cast out demons in your name, work many miracles in your name?' Then I shall tell them to their faces: I have never known you; away from me you evil men!
>
> (Matt. 7:21–3)

Many churches today, far from discerning the dangers of the counterfeit and ruthlessly eradicating it, affirm everything abnormal to be of the Spirit! Christ warned against this: 'False Christs and false prophets will appear and perform great signs and miracles to deceive even the elect . . .' (Matt. 24:24, Mark 13:22).

This must not be dismissed as an isolated expression of rhetoric.

The *problem of deception* is an acute one for most New Testament writers (e.g. 2 Cor. 11:13, Gal. 6:7, Eph. 5:6, 2 Thess. 2:3,9, 2 Pet. 2:1, 1 John 4:1, Rev. 20:3,7,10).

Paul warned the Thessalonians that the work of Satan will display 'all kinds of counterfeit miracles, signs and wonders' (2 Thess. 2:9), and when he encountered counterfeit prophecy he exorcized the slave girl responsible at quite enormous cost to himself and his ministry (Acts 16:16–24).

Today there are many church fellowships that have been torn apart by the infiltration of power-hungry wonder-workers who seem to minister impressively in the name of Christ. Great care must be exercised with such people.

Simon Magus

Simon's story ought to be compulsory reading for all those engaged in the healing ministry!

He had a cult following even in the third century such was the impact he made on Samaria. According to Acts 8:9ff he amazed all classes who gave him their attention. They exclaimed, 'He is the divine power that is called Great!'

Simon believed the gospel and was baptized. He then followed Philip everywhere, amazed at the wonders and miracles of his ministry. Then Peter and John arrived and prayed for the baptized Samaritans that they might receive the Holy Spirit. When Simon saw the remarkable results he offered the Apostles cash for the same gift!

Peter gave Simon a real earful!

'To hell with you and your money!' is J. B. Phillips' accurate translation of Peter's less than encouraging response!

> . . . for thinking that money could buy what God has given for nothing! You have no share, no right, in this; God can see how your heart is warped. Repent of this wickedness of yours, and pray to the Lord that you may be forgiven for thinking as you did; it is plain to me that you are trapped in the bitterness of gall and the chains of sin. (8:20–3)

Simon had responded to the gospel, had believed, and had been baptized. He was a person of immense influence and a full member of the Christian community who kept close company with its leader. Yet, like many today, he felt that no break with his past life was necessary and in ignorance infiltrated and tarnished the church with his paganism and occultism. Often miracles of magic are much more impressive than miracles of faith, and his wonders might well have outshone those of Philip. Might Philip have invited him to minister at his next public healing service!?

When Simon disappears from the pages of the New Testament his last act is (significantly) not to pray himself but to ask Peter to pray for him that what he had predicted would not come to pass.

Other ancient literature continues Simon's story. He claimed to the Samaritans that he was God the Father, to the Jews that he was Jesus Christ (who had not actually suffered), and to the world that he was the Holy Spirit! He thought that by rising again after three days' burial he would demonstrate that he was divine!

He didn't; and wasn't!

In your Name!

At Ephesus, where Paul had healed so many (Acts 19:11–12), seven brothers tried to exorcize in the Name of Christ. But the use of Christ's Name (as Christ himself warned (Matt. 7:22–3)) does not necessarily indicate any spiritual identification with him. The evil spirit replied, 'Jesus I recognize, and I know who Paul is, but who are you?' The demoniac overpowered them so that they fled the house naked and bleeding (Acts 19:13–16)!

This incident led to the pagan wonder-workers of the town burning their precious books of magic at the combined cost of over a hundred years' wages (19:18–20).

If there *was* a shift in the New Testament church from 'charismatic' towards the 'sacramental' ministry, then the likely reasons are the age-old problems of the *ambiguity of wonders* and the *dangers of deception*.

This is an important warning (regardless of its relevance or otherwise to New Testament practice). The supernatural is not necessarily Christian – and there is the devil to prove it! The majority of wonder-working is not the Holy Spirit. Extreme care – and sometimes extreme measures – are necessary to protect the faithful from indiscriminately following every wonder-worker who uses the Name of Christ or heals in his Name.

General Healings in the New Testament

Although the individual stories of healing form some basis for study they are far from the whole story. The individual incidents are backed up, in the Gospels and Acts, by no less than *eighteen* records of general or group healings. These add very considerable weight to the evidence for healing.

Of the twelve group healings in the Gospels, Matthew records all but one of them (4:23–5, 8:16–17, 9:35, 11:1–6, 12:15–16, 13:58 (see Mark 6:5), 14:14, 35–6, 15:30–1, 19:2, 21:14) and Luke provides the twelfth (5:15). Exorcism is mentioned in a third of the accounts, but none mention raising the dead.

When individual incidents and group ministries

are taken together, the Gospels furnish us with *thirty-eight* different instances.

In the Acts there are *eight* mentions of general healing ministry (2:43*, 5:12*, 5:15–16, 6:8*, 8:6–7, 14:3*, 19:11–12, 28:9). Those marked with an asterisk are occasions when 'signs and wonders' took place. (I assume from the accounts of apostolic ministry elsewhere that these will have included healings. To believe that on these four occasions they ignored the sick to walk on water, blast fig trees, and change water into wine, is a less probable assumption than my own!)

The ministers of these group healings are, respectively: the Apostles; the Apostles; Peter; Stephen; Philip; Paul and Barnabas; Paul; Paul.

The witness of such widespread ministry to groups goes some considerable way towards the justification of healing services; although spontaneous ministry to the gathered is not the same as planned ministry to the invited.

Health and Salvation

Even more important for our thinking about public healing services is the New Testament view of 'health'. It is far, far greater than ours. The Greek word *sozo*, for instance, is used for the healing of man's whole being; body, soul and spirit. English has no equivalent word unless we extend the use of *healing* way beyond that of merely physical recovery. This is in keeping with current views of 'health' which are now invariably not only to do with personal wholeness but also right-relationship to society and environment.

Bishop Michael Marshall, in a lecture to the Guild

51

of St Raphael, claimed that in the New Testament 'healing' and 'salvation' were virtually interchangeable terms.[2] The same basic word is used, for instance, of the physical healing of a leper (Luke 17:19), of the spiritual deliverance of a demoniac (Luke 8:36), and of the healing transformation of Zacchaeus and his household (Luke 19:9). The translation by Tyndale (d. 1536) of Jesus's words to Zacchaeus have often been noted and quoted – '*Today health has come to this house*'.

To heal *in the Name of Jesus* takes on a deeper meaning when, as Lord Coggan pointed out in a seminal essay on healing some years ago[3] his very *name* means to *save*! The great Biblical word *shalom*, 'peace', designates being whole. Dr Wilkinson, whose important book I have already commended, summarizes the New Testament view of 'health' as *life, blessedness, holiness* and *maturity*.

The familiar stories of individual healings often express this. Nine lepers were merely 'cleansed', only the one who turned again to Jesus and gave thanks (Gk: *eucharist*) and glorified God was *healed/saved* (Luke 17:14–19). The paralytic at Capernaum was not only cured but forgiven (Mark 2:1–12). Legion sat, clothed and in his right mind, and longed to follow Jesus (Luke 8:38). It is surely a happy *double entendre* that Bartimaeus 'followed Jesus in the *way*' (Mark 10:52, see also John 14:6, Acts 9:2). Peter's mother-in-law immediately served others when healed (Mark 1:31). The woman in the crowd is not merely cured but moved into a new life of 'shalom'/peace (Mark 5:34).

When Peter and John healed the lame man at the Gate Beautiful, he was not simply cured, but entered right into the life/blessedness/holiness/maturity of New Testament *health*. ' . . . He jumped up, stood, and began to walk, and went with them into the Temple, walking and jumping and praising God' (Acts 3:8). True Gospel-health always multiplies. Gospel begets gospel! For

> Everyone could see him walking and praising God, and they recognised him that used to sit begging . . .
> They were astonished and unable to explain what had happened . . .
> Everyone came running towards them . . .
> Peter saw the people and addressed them . . .
> ' . . . God raised him [Jesus] from the dead . . .
> It is faith in that name that has restored this man to health.'
> . . . They were baptised . . . and three thousand were added to their number. (Acts 3:9ff)

To reflect on Acts 3—4 is a worthwhile exercise in relation to the healing ministry. It begins with Peter *having spiritual authority but lacking financial security*. If churches are failing to bring health it may be because most of them have reversed this – and opted for *financial security at the expense of spiritual authority*. (This is usually true even of those who boast of 'Apostolic Succession'.)

The healing of the cripple resulted both in a persecution (4:1ff) and a pentecost (4:31).

The complete story gives us a fair picture of the change and challenge, the comfort and the cost we encounter if we dare to invite the healing Christ.

1. Quoted in *The Apocryphal New Testament*, M. R. James, Oxford.

2. 'The Person of Christ and the Power of Healing' (tape).
3. 'The Ministry of Healing', in *Convictions*, Hodder.

5

Questioning

It is wise to tackle certain basic questions before
embarking on healing services. I shall now turn to
the following:
1. Can healing services be justified?
2. If so, what is their relation to medicine?
3. What about motive and aim?
4. What is the role of faith in healing?
5. Can the Laying-on-of-hands be justified today?
What does it mean?
6. What is anointing all about?
Just to have *an* answer to these questions is not
sufficient. We need the right answer as we seek the
mind of the Church. Our ministries are the
outworking of our opinions. If our beliefs are not
firmly founded our ministry to others will not be
sound.

1. Can public healing services be justified?

The following reasons are those most commonly
raised for *not* having such services.
(i) There is no Biblical equivalent.
(ii) Preparation of those present is not possible.
(iii) False hopes must not be raised.
(iv) 'Every service is a healing service.'
(v) 'We mustn't over-emphasize this ministry.'

(vi) The problem of after-care.

These are very real objections, and we may learn much by facing them. Let us consider each in turn.

(i) Biblical Equivalent?

There is no *exact* equivalent to be sure. But there are a number of things that would seem to make them a right development.

The policy of James's teaching (5:13ff) in which the initiative lies with the *sick* to invite the *elders* and not *vice versa*, is not the only principle in the New Testament.

Leaders did, on occasions, take the initiative. Jesus did so with four individuals (Luke 13:12, John 5:6, Luke 22:51, Luke 7:14). He took the initiative in no less than a third of his dozen group ministries. This tendency is even stronger in the Acts. Only once did an individual take the initiative (3:1–10); it was usually taken by others, e.g. Peter (9:34), Ananias (9:17), or Paul (14:9, 16:18, 20:10, 28:8).

The twenty different occasions of public group healing ministry in the New Testament of largely uninstructed crowds suggest that the Church had no hesitation in risking pastoral dangers to meet pastoral *needs*. If it erred it was on the side of caring.

(ii) The Question of Preparation?

The New Testament crowds were unlikely to have been prepared, but the point is important. This anxiety comes mostly from those familiar with full preparation before Anointing, and those who have experienced the casualties of the if-you-have-faith-you'll-be-healed heresy (see below).

This criticism is more valid with 'open' services than those that minister to an instructed fellowship.

In 'open' services much lack of preparation can be largely offset by:

(a) Making an appropriate introduction, and/or

(b) Ensuring the ministry of the Word is appropriate (see chap. 11).

(iii) False Hopes?

Within an instructed fellowship this does not arise. It is a facet of a lack of preparation, which I have dealt with.

Much can be communicated by the style in which things are done. The necessary step to avoid raising 'false hopes' must not subdue the raising of *true* hope.

One difference between 'spiritual healers' and the Christian ministry is that the former tend to be sickness-orientated, while ours is God-orientated. The mind of the Church is quite clear that such ministry should take place in a context of *worship*. This goes a long way to answering how we distinguish between true hopes and false. 'All our hope on God is founded.' Our hope rests on the loving faithfulness of our Father to whom all present come afresh as children.

(iv) 'Every service is a healing service.'

This is a theological truism!

Every encounter with God is, I believe, a healing encounter. Each time I have heard this objection it is by those who appear to be using it as an excuse! It won't wash! It is like saying every Sunday is a day of resurrection, therefore Easter is superfluous; every day Christ wants to be born anew in us, so let's abolish Christmas!

The Church has always helped its members by

focusing different facets of the gospel at different times and places. Not many of us can 'take in' a museum or art gallery in one go, but have to sample and select our way into their treasures. This is a natural learning process and cannot be bypassed.

Since healing is an authentic aspect of the gospel it would seem odd to treat it differently from all others.

In the perfect church salvation/healing would so pervade everything that no 'focus' on salvation/healing would be necessary. Our aim should be to render healing services obsolete by the healing quality of our worship, fellowship and witness. Until that time comes, it is likely that the occasional focus on the healing work of Christ is right and necessary.

(v) 'We must not over-emphasize this ministry.'

This danger must be recognized, but it is no argument against public healing services as such. It is an incentive to get right their frequency and style. To underplay healing is as much a heresy as to overplay it.

When healing is placed within the context of the Eucharist then its right position is assured.

(vi) The Problem of After-care

As with preparation, this is not so much a problem in services for the Christian fellowship. It increases insofar as a public healing service is opened to the public at large.

If services are adequately thought through, well planned and rightly timed, then there is likely to be both the fellowship and the organization to incorporate and uphold those who need further support.

I have included, later, a number of practical

suggestions that can be taken to encourage adequate follow-up and care.

2. Medicine

Some mention has been made of this already (see pp. 22, 24f.) and I would refer you to my pamphlet *Gospel & Medicine*.

There is really no problem!

If there *is*, then it is unlikely that the ministry reflects the mind of the Church.

The Christian affirmation of medicine stems directly from Scripture.

In the Old Testament, as well as detailed laws for hygiene, there are at least *eleven means* of healing mentioned: food, wine, water, oil, bandages, salt, soda, soap, balm, figs and leaves (Ps. 104:14, 104:15, Exod. 15:22–7, Ps. 23:5, Isa. 1:6, 2 Kings 2:19–22, Jer. 2:22, Gen. 37:25, Isa. 38:21, Ezek. 47:12).

Attitudes to physicians varied before Christ's coming. The most positive view comes in Ecclesiasticus 38:1–15, which provided the model for James's important passage (5:13ff).

> Honour the doctor with the honour that is his due . . .
> for he too has been created by the Lord.
> Healing itself comes from the Most High . . .
> The Lord has brought medicines into existence from the earth . . .
> He uses them to heal and relieve pain . . .
> My son, when you are ill, do not be depressed,
> but pray to the Lord and he will heal you.

Christ did not abolish this. He commanded the blind man to *wash* (John 9:7), and that *food* be brought to Jairus's daughter (Mark 5:43). He used *spittle* on one occasion and made a *mud paste* with it on another (Mark 8:23, John 9:6).

He inspired medicine of every later age with his parable of the Good Samaritan, in which he includes three Old Testament means of healing: *wine*, *oil* and *bandages* (Luke 10:29ff).

Christ's attitude differed greatly from a wonder-worker's. He is recorded as *preparing* people for ministry (Mark 7:33, 8:23), and gathering a right *team* (Mark 5:40). He asked the father of the epileptic demoniac about the *duration* of the illness (9:21), and the blind man, on whom he had laid hands, about the *progress* of the healing (Mark 8:23). He often asked searching *questions* of the sufferers themselves (e.g. Mark 5:9, 10:51, John 5:6, Matt. 9:28), and used *things* to assist healing (outlined above). He frequently gave advice and *direction* to the newly-healed (Mark 1:43–4, 2:11, 5:19, 5:43, 7:36, 8:26, Luke 17:14, John 5:14), and personally *followed up* certain cases (John 5:14, 9:35).

Luke, the 'beloved physician' (Col. 4:14), records Christ using the illustration of a physician and identifying closely with it (4:23, 5:31).

It was an appropriate slip for Origen (AD 185–254) to say that Scripture called Jesus 'the Physician', and his own term 'the good Physician' has persisted to this day.

Paul advised Timothy to drink wine rather than (impure) water (1 Tim. 5:23), and the use of oil for anointing (Mark 6:13, James 5:13–16) will probably, at times, have had medical as well as spiritual significance.

There is no Biblical text against medicine. Failed candidates for the post are 2 Chron. 16:12 and Mark

5:26. In the first, King Asa's sin was not in going to physicians but in breaking his covenant to seek God *first*. The second tells of the failure of physicians to cure the woman's haemorrhage. The point is the severity of her illness that Jesus healed, not that either she or we should avoid medicine. Dr Luke did not waste ink in his account telling us that medicine is costly and has its limitations! He was writing *Good* News!

The key passage for our right understanding of the theological position of medicine is John 5:1–17.

The Man at the Pool

The blind, lame and paralyzed used to gather around Jerusalem's Sheep Pool for its healing properties. The water was disturbed from time to time and those first in benefitted.

There is one verse in the account which is sometimes omitted in early manuscripts, suggesting that some scribes had difficulty with it! It is John's profound insight, '*the angel of the Lord came down into the pool, and the water was disturbed*' (v. 4). The truth of this is not likely to rest in the ability of a first-century witness to capture it on videotape were he so equipped. This is not angelology, but *theo*logy! What John is saying is that when Christ was at the Pool *God was actively healing in* TWO *ways*.

1. In Christ God was healing through his Son.
2. In the Pool God was healing through his Creation.

Some are troubled by the fact that Jesus leaves the crowd and just ministers to the one individual. Only if John's point has been completely missed is this a problem!

Jesus ministered to the one person present who –

61

for thirty-eight years – had *not* been able to avail himself of God's healing in the Pool. In leaving the crowd Jesus does not leave them God-forsaken, but leaves them to partake of his Father's 'divine healing' in and through his Creation!

This is not just first-century mythology, but it is highly relevant today. Behind what today would St John have us see the hand or messenger of God? Obviously in all those things of God's creation which bring us health.

The Theology

As Christians we believe in the Father who *creates* us; the Son who *redeems* us, and the Holy Spirit who *sanctifies* us (i.e. makes us 'holy'). These three 'spheres' of action are

CREATION	REDEMPTION SANCTIFICATION

The respective ministries of Medicine and Church may be set out in relation to the above as follows:

MEDICINE	CHURCH

1. *Medicine applies lessons learned from God's Creation.*
2. *The Church mediates God's grace revealed in Redemption and Sanctification.*

There is widespread confusion over this, so note it carefully!

Medicine applies God's Laws of Nature. Since God *sustains* his creation there is a considerable 'divine' element in it, e.g. 'I put the bones together; God joins them.'

Unlike Medicine, the Church's *distinctive* ministry is not repair prior to eternal death, but rescue prior to eternal life! Medicine's ministry says much about our roots and what we are growing away from; the Church's ministry is about our destiny and what we are growing into.

Medicine may fulfil its goals here because it is of Creation and this life; the Church's ministry has the goals of Redemption of which only the first-fruit is tasted here (Rom. 8:22ff). This accounts for the unhealed, and the agony and the ecstacy of true Redemption ministry!

There are some styles of Christian healing ministry that try to avoid its pain and paradox, by turning the 'first fruits' into the guarantee of what is available *now* rather than as 'signs' of what will be. This is generally dubbed 'triumphalism'.

If the Cross is kept central to all thinking on healing such imbalances are short-lived.

Recently the British Medical Association (BMA) have brought the subject of 'Alternative Medicine' to the fore. The Church's Ministry of Healing is not 'alternative'. Years earlier they wrote, 'As man is body, mind and spirit, and health depends on the harmonious functioning of the whole man, the task of medicine and the Church are *inseparable*'.[1] [Italics mine]

3. Motive and Aim

The motive of any ministry to the needy must always be love. The only motive for having a public healing service is our love and care for those who might attend it.

A healing service is not like a Spring fair – to brighten the image or enlarge the purse. It is far too costly to add healing to the agenda just to keep up with the spiritual Joneses, or because it is the latest bandwagon!

Healing services will be arranged well when the motive for having them is right. An uncaring healing service is a contradiction in terms. It is by no means uncommon for Christians to arrange things for the benefit of others while being quite insensitive to their real needs!

The aim of a public healing service is that God would be glorified. That is not sentimental or pious claptrap. It is all too easy to glorify sickness, healers, ministers, the healed, and/or the church!

Healing is more of a by-product than a target. It is a bit like laughter at a good party! If you get things right it will be there, but you cannot produce it to order! If you aim too hard at healing, it will, like sleep and humility, evade you. God's Kingdom brings health, and it comes by our *openness* and our *obedience*. Our openness not to hinder God and our obedience to serve him.

Probably no publication can teach spiritual openness or obedience, but in all aspects of healing ministry they are vital. The reason is simple. *The right thing done at the wrong time does not bring healing*. Imagine a surgeon who met a patient at a bus-stop and, knowing his need for surgery, stuck a knife in him! A similar action done at the right time and the right place would have been a step towards health. At the wrong place and the wrong time it could be fatal!

Knowing how to plan a healing service, how to lay on hands, how to anoint is of no use whatever unless we use that knowledge *in obedience* to the Father.

Although much church life seems to consist of doing our thing our way and hoping for divine approval, in spiritual ministry of any sort that will not do. In spiritual things the only way forward is obediently to do God's thing, for God only knows (literally!) what is best for every individual. We minister better from a life of openness and obedience than by excellent technique and expertise used at the wrong time.

4. The Place of Faith

I have already referred to the 'faith heresy', and the deliberate avoidance of the term 'faith healing' by mainstream churches (pp. 21, 24).

'If you have faith, you will be healed' seems to be the message of a number of healing stories, and is the basis of many influential ministries today. It sounds Biblical enough! Charles Farah deals with this in his excellent book *From the Pinnacle of the Temple*, subtitled: 'Faith or Presumption?'

What do we mean by 'faith' and what is its place in healing?

Scripture Teaching

(i) In the Old Testament 'faith' as a word is rarely used, but man is constantly urged to live a life of faith. God has repeatedly demonstrated that he is faithful and utterly trustworthy. We should trust his promises and obey his commands. This is having 'faith'. Having faith in God means not putting one's faith in man for his might (Isa. 31:1), understanding (Prov. 3:5) or spirituality (Ezek. 33:13). The only object of faith in the Old Testament is God himself (Ps. 18:2).

(ii) When therefore God visits and redeems his

people, so the divine object of faith becomes *Jesus Christ*. He is the one central object of Christian belief and trust, and for centuries Christ's gospel has been called 'the Faith', and his followers 'the Faithful'.

The New Testament words of believing are often followed by *into* Christ, and this Christward movement helps us to understand the faith verses.

Faith is not mentioned at all in twenty-four of the individual healing stories. Sometimes it was not present among the people concerned, e.g. the raising of the widow's son (Luke 7:11–17), and the man at the Pool (John 5:1–17). John never mentions it.

The word 'faith' occurs in less than a third of the accounts of individual healings. (Three of the parallel accounts do not mention it, which shows that it may have been present even when it was not recorded.)

Jesus *noticed* the faith of the paralytic (Mark 2:5), and Paul similarly noticed the cripple's faith at Lystra (Acts 14:9). Jesus *encouraged* the faith of parents in relation to their children's healing (Mark 5:36, 9:24).

Only on three occasions is it in some measure *related* to the degree of healing: the Centurion's servant; the two blind men indoors, and the Syro-Phoenician's daughter (Matt. 8:5–13, 9:27–31, 15:28). Faith *contributes* to the healing of the woman with the haemorrhage, blind Bartimaeus, and the lame man at Gate Beautiful (Mark 5:34, 10:52, Acts 3:16). Peter's words concerning the latter are worth noting. 'By faith in his [Jesus's] name, has made this man strong . . . the faith which is through Jesus has given the man this perfect health' (RSV). The object of faith is *God*, we do not put our faith in healers or in healing!

We can learn a great deal about 'faith' in the gospel healing stories if we first consider what it means to have faith 'in' someone.

I hope you have faith in your family doctor. If you do *not*, you will probably avoid meeting him and ignore his advice!

But if you *have* faith in him you will be willing to (a) meet him, (b) listen to him, and (c) obey him. Such obedience may mean doing things that you neither understand nor enjoy; it may mean agreeing to surgery that frightens you. But such obedience is possible if you have faith in your doctor knowing that all he directs is for your ultimate good.

A doctor will encourage our faith in him and use it. If, however, one day we were to be knocked-for-six by a bus, we might well wake up to find that the doctors and surgeons had cared for us without either our consent or knowledge!

Their care of us will not have been dependent on the measure of our trust or faith in them. Our faith does not increase their care, but it will probably enable us to benefit most from the care that is given.

If we have no faith in a doctor we will neither summon him nor visit him. *Faith brings us to the healer*, and when there, enables us to *listen* and to *obey*.

The hallmark of 'faith' is *obedience*. With the exception of healing at a distance, in all the 'faith' stories of healing in the New Testament obedience is required and explicit.

Faith in healing is not, as some seem to think, a spiritual pressure we can bring to bear on God to guarantee that he conforms to our will. It is a spiritual grace given us whereby we are drawn to Christ, enabled to trust him, and are willing to conform to his will. For, as St Bernard said, it is when we are conformed that we are transformed.

I have dealt with the first four basic questions that need to be considered before healing services are embarked upon – their justification; their relationship to medicine; our purpose; and the role of faith.

In the next two chapters I shall tackle the remaining two topics – the Laying-on-of-hands and Anointing.

1. Quoted in my *But Deliver Us From Evil*, p. 6.

6

Touching

The Laying-on-of-hands is one of the most usual items of healing services. There has been a great increase of it in recent years, but little attention has been given to its meaning, symbolism or practice.

It is commonly held that it is essentially about some transfer of healing power by those who have an invisible form of healing or spiritual energy.

Francis MacNutt for instance quotes the scientifically demonstrated fact that the growth of seedlings can be accelerated by having hands laid over them, as if it were relevant. Popular magazines regularly have examples of Kirlian photography that show the fingers of healers radiating 'flames' of energy like adverts for high speed gas!

Spiritualists and others hold hands in a circle to create a psychic 'battery' of power into which the sick may plug! This is nothing new, and each generation has shown interest in these invisible forces, and named and renamed them – 'life force', 'prana', 'odic force', 'orgone energy', 'para-electricity', 'bioplasma' and so on.

There have always been a few who believe that the Church's Healing Ministry can be accounted for by such forces and promoted by understanding and tapping them.

There is some reference in Christ's ministry to them. Crowds came to him for healing because, as

Luke particularly points out (6:19, cf. Mark 3:10), 'power came out of him'.

In the better known incident of the woman in the crowd, she believed she would be cured if she but touched his garments (Mark 5:28). I shall elaborate this story later (see chapter 11). Suffice it here to point out that Christ *corrected* her false impression by teaching that the basis of the cure was not her physical contact with him but in her spiritual relationship to him, i.e. her 'faith' (Mark 5:34). It was her faith that made the healing encounter possible. Faith may be likened to the taxi that takes us to the hospital! The taxi does not cure us, but it may well make the cure possible.

A nun once wrote to me saying that she experienced warmth in her hands when she prayed over people. She concluded, wrongly, that this indicated that she had the Christian charism of healing. While this gift may sometimes be accompanied by warmth, tingling, cold, and so on, such manifestations are just human, and accompany the ministry of non-Christians.

Such phenomena have no religious significance, and it is highly dangerous to base anything on them. To assume that because something is *invisible* it is therefore *spiritual*, and because it is 'spiritual' that it is therefore of the *Holy Spirit* is a folly. (Such a formula makes even the devil divine, but it is regularly perpetrated!)

The invisible world is a hotchpotch, ranging from the divine to the demonic – and all stations in between! St John of the Cross and others warn us of the ambiguity of all such things. Warmths, tinglings, vibrations are no more spiritual than hiccoughs – and are best thought of in the same way as meaningless quirks of humanity that are a little embarrassing and should not be encouraged!

In my pamphlet *Laying on of Hands* I tell of a Christian woman – who probably regarded herself as God's gift to the healing ministry! She was standing in a pub with a cigarette in one hand and a drink in the other. A man present complained of asthma. She felt he needed the Laying-on-of-hands, so without putting down either her cigarette or drink she continued the conversation she was having and touched the asthmatic on the chest!!

Actions speak louder than words. As wrong words deceive and lie, so wrong actions do so even more loudly! I am sure her intention was to heal, and at least she responded to human need rather than ignored it.

Her grotesque behaviour demonstrates the necessity for us to understand the Laying-on-of-hands and to minister it in a style that is theologically true and pastorally appropriate in any given situation.

As with all pastoral activities there is no one 'correct' way to minister the Laying-on-of-hands. Just as the administration of the Eucharist in a cathedral will differ from its style in an intensive care unit, so what matters most is not correctness but *appropriateness*.

What was wrong with the behaviour of the woman in the pub was that it was wholly inappropriate. Her wrong actions told loud lies about the source of the blessing, about God's relationship to the sufferer, and about the sufferer's worth.

Such foolishness arises from a basic failure to understand what the Laying-on-of-hands *is* in Christian ministry. To learn this we need to look firstly at Scripture.

Scripture

Surprisingly there is no account of the Laying-on-of-hands in the Old Testament being given for healing. But in writing that I am, perhaps, being too narrow in my classification of 'healing'.

It is certainly used in *blessing*. Israel blesses his grandchildren by the Laying-on-of-hands (Gen. 48:14ff). When a group was blessed and individual Laying-on-of-hands was impractical, Aaron 'raised his hands towards the people and blessed them' (Lev. 9:22). (Such a style of group blessing is usual today at the conclusion of most Christian worship.)

When God appoints Joshua, Moses expresses this *commission* by laying hands on him (Num. 27:16ff).

The well-known Aaronic blessing reminds us that it is God who blesses:

The Lord bless you and keep you,
The Lord cause his face to shine upon you . . .

(Num. 6:24ff)

We can neither bless, commission, nor heal. These are the actions of God which we may be called to symbolize.

The Laying-on-of-hands in the Old Testament is used in dedication, in sacrifice and with capital offenders. (These other usages I have outlined in my pamphlet *Laying on of hands* and they need not concern us here. They do not express God's action man-ward, as in blessing/commissioning/healing, but rather man's action Godward or outward.)

The distinction between God's action man-ward and man's action Godward is important. The people laid hands on the Levites to dedicate them *to God* (Num. 8:10–12). It was a Godward act done by the people not the priests. It does not give any Biblical basis for the laity ministering the Laying-on-of-hands to bless or heal, since the 'direction' of blessing/healing is God man-ward, not man Godward. (I am not saying that the laity should not do this, simply that the people laying hands on the Levites provides no precedent.)

Touch, but not the formal Laying-on-of-hands, was used in healing. Elijah stretched himself three times upon the widow's dead child (1 Kings 17:21ff) as did Elisha upon the Shunammite lad (2 Kings 4:32ff). An accidental touch of Elisha's dead bones restored a corpse to life according to 2 Kings 13:21 – an odd event which may not be totally unrelated to the history of healing shrines.

New Testament

As in the Old Testament era, hands are laid on for *blessing* and *commissioning*.

Jesus blessed the children (Matt. 19:13), and the accounts of the Ascension tell of Christ blessing a gathering, as Aaron had done, by *lifting up his hands* (Luke 24:50).

In addition, the imposition of hands was used for *Initiation* and the *Giving of the Spirit* (Acts 8:14ff, 19:2ff, 9:12–20, cf. also Heb. 6:2, and 1 Tim. 5:22).

Ananias laid hands on Saul for him to be filled with the Holy Spirit and for *healing* (Acts 9:17), and did so standing (Acts 22:13). Ananias was, note, not an Apostle but, in modern terms, a layman. (To suggest, as F. F. Bruce does, that on that particular occasion he was a 'duly commissioned apostle' is to impose twentieth-century theological order upon the variety of first-century pastoral practice!)

The majority of the New Testament references

are, of course, for healing, and the Laying-on-of-hands for this purpose is never man-God-ward but always God-man-ward. Expressed in spatial terms, it is 'downward', and the standing of Ananias and the authoritative 'praying *over*' individuals (James 5:14) is surely related to this.

I personally think it helpful not to distinguish rigidly between the Laying-on-of-hands to *bless* and to *heal*, but to regard 'healing' as the *blessing of the sick*. Any sick person who is blessed will hope that it results in healing!

Our Lord's practice varied enormously because he always ministered *appropriately*.

In half of the twenty-six recorded incidents of his individual healings no mention is made of touch or the Laying-on-of-hands. But of these, five were demoniacs whom Jesus never seems to have touched, and three were at a distance.

Jesus's use of touch or the Laying-on-of-hands can be roughly summarized as follows:

1. Taking by the Hand

This he did according to the earliest account with Peter's mother-in-law (Mark 1:31, cf. Matt. 8:15), and in all three accounts of Jairus's daughter (Mark 5:41, etc.). The epileptic demoniac was raised up in this way after the exorcism (Mark 9:27).

2. Touching the Afflicted Area

(a) MEDICALLY

Christ put a mud-paste on the eyes of the man at the Pool (John 9:6), and saliva on the eyes of the blind man at Bethsaida (Mark 8:23). He may also have used saliva when healing the deaf mute; the text is unclear (Mark 7:33–4).

(b) NON-MEDICALLY

Christ touched the eyes of the blind man at Bethsaida (Mark 8:25), and, according to Matthew, the eyes of Bartimaeus (20:34 cf. Mark 10:46–52), and the two other blind men (9:29). He touched the ear of the injured Malchus (Luke 22:51) and, appropriately, both the ears and tongue of the deaf-mute (Mark 7:33).

3. Touching the Person

Each synoptic Gospel records Jesus touching the leper (Mark 1:41, Matt. 8:3, Luke 5:13).

4. Laying-on-of-hands

The term to 'lay on hands' is used in the healing of the woman bent double (Luke 13:13), and twice in the account of the blind man at Bethsaida (Mark 8:23,25). Luke alone uses it of the evening clinic at Capernaum (4:40), and Mark mentions it in connection with Christ's restricted ministry among the unbelievers of Nazareth (6:5).

Interestingly it was the Laying-on-of-hands that Jairus sought for his daughter (Mark 5:23), and what others wanted for the deaf mute (Mark 7:32). Jesus's response to the requests was not exactly as either expected. By the time he reached Jairus's daughter she was dead, and a raising rather than a healing was necessary.

With the man who could neither hear nor speak Jesus did not simply lay on hands, but instead engaged in an elaborate six-part mime of indicating, spitting, touching, looking, sighing and speaking to convey what he was doing (Mark 7:33–4).

5. Conclusions

What can be noted from Christ's own ministry?

The Laying-on-of-hands was not Christ's most usual method of healing. More often he healed by the *word* spoken. Of the individual healings recorded in Scripture, touch or the Laying-on-of-hands accompanied only about a *half* of the healings by authoritative word. There is only one case of touching to heal without accompanying words being recorded. That was the case of Malchus's ear (Luke 22:51) which was cut off in the fracas at Gethsemane. The strange situation may more than explain it!

The accounts are sometimes very short (e.g. Matt. 9:33), and it is risky to argue from silence. The following may be fairly deduced from our Lord's own ministry.

(i) Touch or the Laying-on-of-hands when used accompanied the healing word.

(ii) It was not necessary. Christ usually healed without it.

(iii) He seems not to have touched demoniacs. The most obvious reason is that touch reinforces our relationship to the other *person*. But the words of exorcism are not addressed to the person who can be touched, but to the invading spiritual forces. To touch the *person* while addressing the *evil* tends to confuse rather than clarify what is going on.

(iv) Christ showed great flexibility and adaptability. Even identical symptoms were not ministered to uniformly.

(v) When appropriate he touched the ritually unclean like the leper and Jairus's dead daughter

(Mark 1:41, 5:41), and ignored the ritual implications (Num. 19:11–13), but regarded uncleanness as moral and spiritual rather than physical in origin (Mark 7:1–23).

(vi) He was willing to take the initiative (Luke 14:4, 22:51, Mark 6:5) but readily responded to cries for mercy (Matt. 9:27, 15:22, Mark 9:22, 10:47, Luke 17:13).

(vii) His compassion was noted (Mark 1:41, Luke 7:13, Matt. 20:34).

When we turn from the ministry of Jesus himself to that of the Apostolic Church much the same patterns are apparent.

In eight individual healings (I include raisings and exorcism) of Acts, touch and the Laying-on-of-hands continue to be subordinate to the word.

Peter took the lame man by the hand to raise him up (Acts 3:7), while Ananias laid hands on Saul to heal his blindness (9:12,17). Paul laid hands on Publius's sick father (28:8), but did not touch the demoniac girl (16:16–18). The Apostles frequently took the initiative (9:34, 14:9, 16:18, 20:10, 28:8).

An interesting addition in these narratives is the specific mention of prayer. Thus Peter first knelt down and prayed before raising Dorcas from the dead (9:40) – as well he might! Peter himself will later have told others of this because he was alone at the time. He may have remembered his failure to exorcize the epileptic demoniac and Christ's explaining the disciples' lack of prayer (Mark 9:29). Paul at Malta ministered to Publius's father 'after prayer' (28:8).

Ministering the Laying-on-of-hands formally

Very little has been written or taught about actually ministering the Laying-on-of-hands, so I shall look at it in detail.

The first distinction to be made is between *formal* and *semi-formal* ministry.

By 'formal' ministry I mean the use of set words only. By 'semi-formal' ministry I mean that in which the ministrants respond to a spoken or known need of the person with personally appropriate prayer. The latter is most common at public healing services.

When 'formal', like the administration of the Communion Bread and Wine, the ministry is more general. The ministrants have little *external* requirement demanded of them other than the ability to minister the right action coupled with the right words.

If *semi*-formal, then we are into something quite different for the ministrant even if it is perceived no differently by the recipient! It requires a very high degree of spiritual sensitivity and awareness, and is totally demanding, for the successions of individual ministries are done extempore.

Although not desirable, one can 'get away' with formal ministry without preparation and almost regardless of one's spiritual state! Not so the semi-formal to which I shall devote a whole chapter later.

Formal Laying-on-of-hands is often given to the young and other non-communicants.

When formality is used rightly it is a great declaration and demonstration of God's sovereignty. Wrongly used it can become trite and meaningless. The individual blessings given by those of the dab-and-mutter school commit the same sin as the woman-in-the-pub (see above p. 71); to express the loving care of God care*lessly* is theologically and pastorally *inappropriate*. Casual blessing tells lies about God, the event, and the person.

In formal ministry great care must be taken not to trivialize the Laying-on-of-hands. How often I have witnessed the Laying-on-of-hands casually given in under three seconds because 'time is short'. The truth is not that the time is short at all, but that the time is being mismanaged! Children in particular suffer from this. This is particularly sad because the Laying-on-of-hands in blessing on children in adult worship is the natural way in which they are introduced to the healing ministry. If they are treated as second-rate by us they will not readily believe that they are first-rate to God. (See my pamphlet *Children and the Healing Ministry* for much more material.) Lacking a sacramental theology, their meeting with God will rest on the *quality of their encounter* with us.

Christ taught that what we do or not do to others we do – or not do – to him (Matt. 25:40).

The most effective spur to our right ministering is to imagine that after a service the Risen Lord is waiting to say to you, *'It was I whom you touched and for whom you prayed . . .'*

Aim to do it in such a way that you know he would add ' . . . *and thank you very much indeed!*'

There are various ways in which the hands may be laid. If the person kneels before you and bows his head over-much – the choice is limited! Hats are rarely a problem nowadays. If one appears don't embarrass the person by requiring her to remove it, simply lay hands on her shoulders.

It is difficult, I think, to get the pressure right. It is a purposeful act, not a vague or tentative one, the person should not require faith to know that it is happening! On the other hand there are many common states of illness or weakness where too heavy a hand for too long upon the head is intolerable. If two are ministering together a hand each on the person's head seems natural, with the spare hands perhaps resting gently on a shoulder.

In some cases the additional touching or holding of a person's hand is very appropriate.

The way to hold the head of another for their greatest feeling of security is, as some suggest, to hold it cradled with a hand fore n'aft like holding a rugger ball!! If the primary need is for comfort this may be right, but I react against it since it is not the same style in which the Laying-on-of-hands is given on other occasions. To have the Laying-on-of-hands ministered in the same style for initiation, healing, and commissioning keeps healing related to the whole witness and mission of the Christian life.

If it is visually not clear whether the person is symbolically being healed by Christ or sent out by him (Acts 6:6, 13:3) this is no bad thing, for Christian healing is best understood as equipment for Christian service and witness (Mark 1:31, 5:19).

For those for whom the signing of a cross is meaningful the sign may be traced on their brow with the thumb of one hand. For many this will positively relate to and renew their earlier baptism and/or anointing. If a Trinitarian blessing is given such signing would naturally be done to coincide with the words 'Father . . . Son . . . Spirit'.

Form of Words

In formal usage there may be any appropriate prayer and/or blessing. The ministers should know the words by heart. Here are some suggestions.

(i) 'The Touch of Christ.' I introduced this about ten years ago for use in Eucharistic settings where 'The Body of Christ' and 'The Blood of Christ' were used. It has the merits, in that setting, of being clearly sacramental and linked closely to the Communion. It avoids individualism. It has strong Scriptural overtones, and is widely used. (It is so obvious that many will have discovered it independently.)

(ii) A blessing should be fully Trinitarian. (If there is 'no time for that', get things changed!) Here is an example:

> *May the love of God the Father,*
> *The presence of the Risen Christ,*
> *And the power (and healing) of the Holy Spirit*
> *overflow your heart and your home*
> *this day/night and always.*

This prayer, also mine, has the unexpected word 'overflow'. I believe it begins rightly to indicate the outworking of blessing, and readers can improve on it I am sure.

The phrase 'heart and home' attempts to express Christ's touch upon the real person and the whole person, and that their home (to which most will shortly return) is part of what they offer to Christ and part of what is blessed.

It is not difficult to compose such prayers. At the time of writing this my home parish is planning its first Holy Week penitential service with the Laying-on-of-hands. For this we have together devised a Trinitarian blessing based on God's three-fold work of creation, redemption and sanctification.

> *May the love of the Father remake you*
> *May the Cross of the Lord Jesus redeem you*
> *May the fire of the Holy Spirit renew you.*

If a prayer is to last and to be remembered it has to be firm in its structure, tidy in its form and regular in its beat. (See my pamphlet *Twenty-Four Healing Prayers*.) Jesus regularly taught in this way[1] (e.g. Matt. 7:7–8).

(iii) Paul's prayer in 1 Thess. 5:23 is Scripture's nearest to a definition of health. Variations of it are often used.

> *May the God of peace himself sanctify you wholly*
> *and may your spirit and soul and body*
> *be kept sound and blameless*
> *at the coming of our Lord Jesus Christ.*   (RSV)

(iv) Many denominations adopt the choice of the late George Bennett:

> *The healing mercies of our risen Lord Jesus Christ,*
> *present with us now,*
> *fill your whole being, body, mind, soul and spirit,*
> *and heal you.*
> *May he do away from you all that harms or hurts*
> *you and give you his peace.*

(v) The excellent Methodist leaflet *Services of Healing* has one which is certainly easier to use by heart!

> *May the Lord Jesus*
> *grant you healing and renewal.*
> *Go in peace.*

The briefer the prayer the stronger it has to be. I would strengthen it with the addition of 'Christ' and 'forth' and substitute the static nouns for more active verbs.

> *May the Lord Jesus Christ*
> *heal you and renew you.*
> *Go forth in peace.*

A rich variety of material can be found in John Gunstone's excellent book *Prayers for Healing*.

The Ministers?

As I have already stated, ministering formally with set words is very different indeed from ministering extempore in response to spoken needs. The latter requires very special, but not uncommon, gifts, and should be prepared for.

Who should minister formally?

Scriptural practice is that it is generally the Christian leaders, although the contribution of really obedient lay folk, like Ananias, may be very great.

Church leadership should be involved lest the healing ministry should be presented as something on the fringe of Church life. Invite the bishop or circuit superintendent!

When numbers require it, the ministers for formal Laying-on-of-hands should be the local leader and his or her recognized *spiritual* assistants. I have written 'spiritual' since it is a spiritual ministry. Excellent treasurers and indispensable administrative leaders may not be spiritual leaders.

It is good if those ministering can be both men and women – including younger Christians, and indeed if Medicine can be represented. The advantage of *formal* ministry is that more can do it and do it adequately.

The character and nature of those ministering are important. Folk come for the touch of Christ himself. Although we are all far from Christlike we should at least exclude from symbolizing Christ's Person those whose lives do not build up Christ's

Body. (The principles of 1 Timothy 3:1–13 apply to any spiritual leadership.)

Ministering in *pairs* is a good idea, although less essential than it is for semi-formal ministry. This prevents the needy over-identifying with a 'healing individual', and for the ministrants it is easier. It is good preparation if the ministry later develops into the semi-formal (see chapter 10 below).

Children, especially younger ones, should be ministered to eyeball-to-eyeball! Since most church architecture positions them, if kneeling, at shin level, they should stand. The Jews were right, the essence of blessing is the light of God's countenance shining upon us and giving us peace. We should reflect that. Ideally they should be addressed by name.

One vicar whom I served used to minister thus to children at the Eucharist. Crouching to address them face-to-face he would say, 'Hello! What's your name?' Child or parent would reply. 'We're going to ask Jesus to bless you. Would you like that?' The child would generally nod. Then would follow a full Trinitarian blessing. Sound practice! If adults feel it right to deprive children at Communion of what they themselves receive they at least owe it to them to ensure that God's blessing is not experienced as a negative one of brief casual encounter and deprivation. Only a generous personal ministry is theologically sound and pastorally appropriate.

When mothers-to-be come for blessing, it is usual to add a special prayer or blessing for the unborn child.

Provision should always be made to bless in the pew any who are unable to come forward and who desire it. (Future church architecture should ensure that there is at least one wheelchair route to the communion rail.)

I will not give a separate list of guidelines in preparation for *formal* ministry, but will hope that the guidelines for *semi-formal* ministry preparation (with which I conclude this chapter) will be sufficient incentive and inspiration to those with the easier task of ministering formally.

Semi-formal Laying-on-of-hands

Most public healing services have the Laying-on-of-hands in this style. Within the constraints of space and time the aim is to do and say what Christ himself wants said and done. Its hallmark is not *in*formality, but the flexibility to minister *appropriately* to each person. (This may well mean the use of formal prayer if such is the most appropriate.) Sometimes folk will verbalize their need, at other times their words are designed (consciously or unconsciously) to conceal it!

The task is awesome – but don't despair!

Compare it to preaching, for instance. The preacher has *days* to prepare God's *general* word to meet a group's *general* need. He has about twenty minutes in which to do this and delivers it 'six foot above contradiction'!

In semi-formal praying, by contrast, the ministers have *instantly* to convey God's *specific* word to a string of different *specific* personal needs. Each is accomplished in about one minute, and delivered face-to-face!

If preaching normally requires preparation how much more does giving the Touch of Christ in this way?

Preparation

Ideally we should be in such a state of grace that no preparation is necessary. Like marriage, ministering should be approached 'reverently, discreetly, advisedly, soberly and in the fear of God'. For those who would like some suggestions here is a list based on what I would like my own practice to be!

(i) Steep yourself in Scripture. Many appropriate words of ministry will bubble up from this source.

(ii) Experience the Laying-on-of-hands in your own life and know at first hand its repercussions.

(iii) Try to avoid ministering at short notice. A week is ideal. Keep the forthcoming ministry in your prayers.

(iv) As the time approaches try to avoid that which would disturb your peace. Guard against wrong entertainment.

(v) Do not fast on the day, but if possible set aside an earlier day or part day in such preparation.

(vi) Pray daily for the Holy Spirit to shed abroad in your heart God's love for those to whom you will be ministering.

(vii) Pray for the service, its planning, its ministers, those in need, and follow-up.

(viii) Be reconciled and at peace before ministering.

(ix) Use all means of grace available and natural to you to be in spiritually good shape on the day.

(x) Get organized. Arrive early and do not be overtired.

(xi) If ministering in pairs try to ensure that your partner and yourself will work easily and naturally together. (An earlier meeting of 'partners' for sharing and prayer together is a good idea.)

(xii) Submit to the local leadership. Be clear about

the allocation of time. Know what is expected of you – and what not!

A detailed consideration of semi-formal ministry occurs in chapter 12 below.

1. See Dom Robert Petitpierre's *Poems of Jesus*, Faith Press.

7

Oiling

In recent years there has been a considerable shift by many to establish the right use of anointing. The Roman Catholic church has reformed its practice of anointing as a preparation for death, and now anoints for life. Churches in the reformed tradition are recovering from the over-reaction of the seventeenth century Reformers and seeking to be more truly Biblical.

In Christian traditions touched by the charismatic movement there is an increasing appreciation for all that symbolizes or conveys the anointing of the Holy Spirit.

Oil for anointing ought, I think, to be available at every healing service – even if very rarely used. It is lavishly used at some Roman Catholic healing services where they can presume a strong sacramental understanding.

I do not think it would be wise to embark on a healing service without a basic understanding of it. (For a more detailed look at the subject I would refer you to my pamphlet *Understanding Anointing*.)

Anointing

The main thing to grasp is that oil has nothing whatever to do with *sickness*. Why that is so will become clear!

1. Old Testament

In the Old Testament certain people (prophets, priests and kings) and certain things (Temple furnishings) were anointed with oil as an act not of human dedication to God, but God's consecration of a person/thing for himself. Thus the King became known as *God's Anointed One* ('Christ' in Greek).

God's anointing brought with it his Holy Spirit, e.g. upon Moses, Aaron, Saul and others.

God's Chosen People began to realize that in some sense *they* were God's anointed (Hab. 3:13).

2. Oil

Canaan was the 'land of olives' and oil played an important part in the national economy. Solomon's oil exports to Egypt helped to finance his Temple! In Christ's day Herod literally swam in it!

In the home too it was important. It was used for cooking, lighting, washing, and cleansing.

It was so plentiful and was valued so much for its contribution to living that it became a symbol not of sadness but *gladness* (Isa. 61:3). It was for parties, not funerals, and it was frequently linked with *wine*, that other symbol of joy and life.

3. New Testament

Jesus began his public ministry by reading from Isaiah:

> The Spirit of the Lord has been given to me,
> for he has anointed me.
> He has sent me to bring the good news to the poor,
> to proclaim liberty to the captives
> and to give the blind new sight,

to set the downtrodden free,
to proclaim the Lord's year of favour. (Luke 4:18ff)

'This text', he added, 'is being fulfilled today . . .' In other words 'I *am* God's Anointed One, the *Christ*.'

Simon Peter was the first to recognize Jesus as God's Anointed (Mark 8:29), and later, when preaching to the Gentiles (Acts 10:38), he used the same passage when he told how

> God anointed Jesus of Nazareth with the Holy Spirit and with power; and how he went about doing good and healing all who were oppressed by the devil, for God was with him (RSV).

Christ's disciples not only *followed* God's Anointed, but were incorporated *into him* by baptism. Hence Paul speaks of God's people, the Church, sharing Christ's anointing,

> Remember it is God himself who assured us all, and you of our standing in Christ (Gk. *Chris-tos*), and has anointed us (Gk. *Chris-as*), marking us with his seal, and giving us the pledge, the Spirit . . . (2 Cor. 1:21–2).

The followers of the Christ were first called *Christ*-ians at Antioch, and by AD 180 Theophilus of Antioch wrote, 'We are called Christ-ians on this account, because we are anointed with the oil of God.'

It was natural, therefore, for the early Christians to use *oil* in Christian initiation. In some ways it was more appropriate than water which symbolized the washing of the old life, while oil signified the new life in God's Anointed. Oil was soon used in *Christ*-ian marriage, ordination, and coronation.

In 1 Pet. 2:9–10 there is a fine description of *Christ*-ians:

> But you are a chosen race, a royal priesthood, a consecrated nation, a people set apart to sing the praises of God who called you out of darkness into his wonderful light . . . once you were outside the mercy, now you have been given mercy.

'Chosen . . . royal . . . consecrated . . . set-apart' is a concise summary of the meaning of anointing. (The link with 'mercy' is not obvious in English, but in the Greek the words for 'mercy' and 'oil' sound almost the same.)

Oil is, as I stated at the beginning of this section, nothing to do with sickness. Theologically it is about:

The calling of the Father

The coming of the Christ

The empowering of the Holy Spirit.

In Christ the Anointed One has come. At Pentecost his anointing Spirit is poured out to anoint God's people in consecration and in power.

The Apostles anointed the sick in obedience to Christ's command to heal them (Mark 6:12–13). Many cannot understand why the disciples anointed but Christ himself did not. The obvious answer is that where God's Anointed was himself present, that which symbolized him was rendered superfluous. Why be reading the article on royalty if you could be shaking hands with the Queen in person?

Symbols are useful to represent the invisible. In Christ's visible absence it makes sense to use oil. When in Galilee he was visibly present what would oil have added to the event?

The key New Testament passage is in James 5:13–16, in which sick Christians are instructed thus:

91

. . . send for the elders of the church, and they must anoint him with oil in the name of the Lord and pray over him. The prayer of faith will save the sick man and the Lord will raise him up again; and if he has committed any sins, he will be forgiven. So confess your sins to one another, and pray for one another and this will cure you . . .

The early Christians anointed liberally. Relations would anoint the sick all over daily for a week! It was generous and joyful – and rightly so for oil then symbolized just those things!

Oil is not about sickness, but about Life. It is not about us or our maladies but about God's Anointed and his anointing Spirit.

In anointing a sick person we do not give them something abnormal and extraordinary because they are ill. It is the *illness* which is to be regarded as abnormal, not the anointing!

Anointing is according to James and all later Christian practice, a ministry to *Christ*-ians. They are, to coin a phrase, *re-Christ-ed*. Their unity with and in God's Anointed Christ is re-established, re-expressed, reaffirmed and renewed. Perhaps it is the most specifically *Christian* action that can be performed. It is inappropriate to anoint a non-Christian unless it marks a turning to God's Anointed.

It is not surprising that Christians of all streams are wanting to rediscover the right contemporary use of this great Christian symbol in initiation and healing.

In the early church the laity used to anoint, but because some regarded the oil as magical and divorced from prayer, the Church later restricted its use to priests. Modern understanding has sought to rediscover a fuller use of oil. The Roman Catholics

Francis MacNutt and Barbara Shlemon both advocate the use of oil by laity, in their respective books *The Power to Heal* and *To Heal as Jesus Healed*.

Certain points in James's teaching about anointing should be noted for guidance.

(i) It concerns the Christian sick.

(ii) They summon the elders.

(iii) Their task is essentially spiritual, not psychiatric, medical or social. They are to anoint and pray.

(iv) The sick person will be saved/healed.

(v) God will use faithful prayer in bringing this about.

(vi) God will raise up the sick.

(vii) His/her sins will be forgiven.

(viii) We are to confess our sins to one another, and

(ix) pray for each other so that we too may be cured. (An exposition of this would take another book!)

James's teaching is very up-to-date in its *corporate* concept both of sin and healing, and also in the healing importance he places on confession of sin.

The summoning of the elders was done immediately and once only. (This is the implication of the changed tense of the Greek verb according to Dr John Wilkinson whose book I have already commended.)

The passage promotes the use of oil, but does not attribute healing properties to it. James thus avoids the pitfall of magical thinking. It is in the *spiritual* realm, in the prayer of faith, and in the Lord's own action, that the causes of healing are to be found. (James would never have guessed the later tendency of Christians to think magically about spiritual things as well!)

The recovery word used is 'save' (see above pp. 51–3), so healing is placed within the salvation programme of God. Linked to this is the fact that the sick person does not get up but is *raised up*. The overtones of resurrection are obvious and deliberate. (The same word is used of the resurrection in e.g. Matt. 16:21, Mark 16:6, Luke 24:34, and Acts 5:30.)

The confession of sin is, surprisingly, not to the elders, but to 'one another'. This mutual ministry, with prayer, is regarded as a characteristic of the community.

4. Ministering Unction

It is beyond the scope of this book to spell out how anointing takes place outside of a public healing service. But in relation to public healing services it is relevant to note that:

(i) It is administered only to the Christian sick.

(ii) It is usually only administered once per illness. (The Laying-on-of-hands may be used after anointing as a regular and sustaining ministry.)

(iii) The person concerned is always prepared beforehand and as part of this is usually asked to review his or her life, and to request spiritual direction and other ministry if appropriate.

(iv) Except in an emergency it takes place within a Eucharist, and is accompanied by the Laying-on-of-hands.

These points indicate why it is not often used in public healing services, but real divine guidance and pastoral sensitivity require on occasions the bending, if not breaking, of our 'rules'. Where the Lord is really 'present to heal' then there is often a concertina-ing of processes which are more usually spaced out. (When miracles occur they are often a concertina-ing of events which would be generally expected to take place over a far greater period.)

We must be sensitive and alert to those special

occasions when divine grace is flowing freely. Conferences and retreats where the Christian fellowship, prayer and expectancy deepen over three or four days are sometimes occasions in a totally different league, spiritually, from that sustained locally by an hour a week.

Although healing services are brief, our prayers should do much to make them different. If those attending are really prayed for earlier by the local Christians, then a *divinely initiated and guided preparation* will have been going on long before the actual service – perhaps even before we had ever thought of having one!

The oil used is generally pure olive oil. In episcopal denominations the bishop blesses the oils on Maundy Thursday for the use of his clergy in their ministry. I heartily commend this practice in principle to Christians of non-episcopal traditions. I do not do so because the oil so blessed is any more 'powerful', but it is a great encouragement to the sick (who invariably feel isolated and lonely) to feel, by such symbolism, that they matter and are cared for not just by their friends, but by the wider Church.

When the oil is blessed by the area's Christian leader it places the practice of anointing at the centre of Church life and witness. It dispels fears that the practice and its practitioners are odd!

Those who have inherited no tradition in these matters tend to read James, buy some oil, pray and pour it over the person's head.

Traditionally, anointing is done much more sparingly by dipping a thumb in the oil and by tracing on the forehead of the person concerned the sign of the Cross. The forehead indicates that it is the sick *person*, not just the afflicted part, that is the object of God's blessing. Even the custom in some traditions of anointing the five senses retains this.

Since the sign of the Cross is the most Christian symbol that exists do not hesitate to use it. Let us not be dominated by past allergies to the practices of other Christians. (If the sign of the Cross is a good thing to put on a church gate or church lampshade why deprive the sick of it?)

The oil has, traditionally, always been conscientiously removed with cotton wool. This is totally *inappropriate* and is theological, psychological and pastoral nonsense! If it is a good symbol to *apply*, it cannot also be a good symbol to *remove*! It remains a symbol after the service. Use it sparingly and *leave it* (like the imposition of ashes that some readers will be familiar with).

At a public healing service local ministers may prepare their sick folk and arrange for them to come for anointing.

When administered privately the form of words can easily be taken from a book. At a public healing service, if oil is made available, then a card with an appropriate prayer on it needs to be at hand also. One form runs:

[Name] I anoint you with oil in the name of our Lord Jesus Christ. May our heavenly Father make you whole in body and mind, and grant you the inward anointing of his Holy Spirit, the Spirit of strength and joy and peace.

In the 1935 service (see above p. 17) the anointing is sandwiched between two prayers. The first asks for God's help and goodness to be shown to the sufferer for his or her healing and restoration. Both prayers are accompanied by the Laying-on-of-hands. The second prayer is so fine, that I shall quote it in full (while taking the liberty, fifty years on, of changing the 'thees' to 'yous', and 'Ghost' to 'Spirit').

> As with this visible oil your body is outwardly anointed, so may our heavenly Father grant of his infinite goodness that your soul may be inwardly anointed with the Holy Spirit, and filled with strength and comfort.
> May the almighty God restore to you (bodily) health and strength to serve him.
> May he send to you freedom from all your pains, troubles and diseases, whether of body or mind.
> May he pardon you all your sins and offences; and grant you strength to serve him truly; that aided by his Holy Spirit, you may have perfect victory and triumph over Satan, sin, disease, and death; through Jesus Christ our Lord, who by his death has destroyed death, and now with the Father and the Holy Spirit evermore lives and reigns, God, world without end. Amen.

No wonder the sick recover! What an antidote to our fashionable spiritual anaemia that we peddle in an attempt to sell our faith and make it easy!

Over twenty-five years ago I was with my crippled mother when she was anointed. After the service (a home one) while I was still kneeling, she got up and walked! She was instantly and lastingly healed.

Whenever I have had the privilege of anointing another, the use of such a prayer as the above certainly strengthens *me*!

The use of what might be called an 'external' form of words is often stronger, richer and more balanced than most of us could produce extempore. It has the added advantage of saving the minister from the strain of discerning what he ought to say and how to say it.

There is a certain authority in using something greater than our merely individual repertoire. It reinforces the important conviction that the healing ministry is truly the healing ministry of the *Church*.

If we follow too much the fashion of being *personal* above all else, we may appeal more to some but long-term there is a real danger that their spiritual diet will shrink to our size. Liberty should result in enrichment not malnutrition!

The practice of anointing in initiation and for healing is growing and is unlikely to diminish. While many sufferers appreciate being the focus of the church's prayers there are few who enjoy being the focus of the church's attention!

If any sick are anointed publicly one way which gives the event some 'size' while keeping the ministry itself appropriate to the individual is to have the congregation sing about it!

The following hymn is the only one to date that I know of which is based on the anointing teaching of James 5:13ff.

1. Father, sending Your Anointed
   Son to save, forgive, and heal,
   And, through Him, Your Holy Spirit
   To make our salvation real;
2. Look upon our ills and trouble
   And on those who suffer much.
   Send Your church the Spirit's unction
   In Christ's Name to heal and touch.
3. Grant forgiveness to the faithful;
   Bring to unity their prayer,
   Use it for Your work unhindered
   Through both sacrament and care.

4.*May the one/ones to be anointed
   Outwardly with oil this hour,
   Know Christ's fullest restoration
   Through the Holy Spirit's power.
5. Heal Your church. Anoint and send us
   Out into the world to tell
   Of your love and blessings to us;
   How, in Christ, 'All will be well.'†
(From *Mission Praise 2*, (c) J. Richards)

---

* Optional verse for when anointing takes place.
† Metre 8.7.8.7. Suggested tune: *St Andrew*.

8

Deciding

Now we know what it is all about we can start making some decisions!

The main questions are these. I shall later comment on each.

(i) Is a good healing service right in principle?

(ii) If right in principle is it appropriate to consider having one in *this* situation?

(iii) If 'yes', then is it to be a one-church affair?

(iv) Should it be ecumenical?

(v) Is its main aim exclusively to build up the faithful?

(vi) Is one aim to give some public witness to the words and works of the gospel?

(vii) Depending on some earlier answers is it appropriate to be Eucharist-based or not?

(viii) Is the event a once-off or is it to initiate something regular?

Here are some reflections on these issues.

1. Right in Principle?

I believe that public healing services are only right in principle if they are *good ones*. I mean by that that they are only right *if* they reflect the mind of the Church in such matters as health, medicine, faith and so on.

It is not my purpose in this book to encourage

healing services just for the sake of it, but to encourage *good ones* as and when *appropriate*.

The mind of the Church is clearly that they *do* have a place within its total life and witness. They are right in principle but in practice they need to be based on firm foundations and balanced teaching if they are to enrich church life rather than distort it. (That is why I have taken seven chapters to reach this point!)

2. Right in this Situation?

One of the characteristics of the healing ministry is that in bringing God, as it were, 'closer', people become threatened. Healing upsets the status quo. It is only Good News to some, to others it is bad! The Scriptures repeatedly bear this out.

Mary's Magnificat was good news to the hungry and those of low degree, but bad news to the mighty and the rich (Luke 1:52–3).

The transformation of the gospel regularly brings both rejoicing and anger. In the healing of the mad 'Legion', the story ends with the mad made sane and the sane becoming mad! For Legion is sitting, sane, and wanting to follow Jesus, while the 'normal' pig-farmers become mad enough to want to drive away the Great Physician (Mark 5:15–18)!

This is no isolated incident. In the long account in John's Gospel of the man born blind, *no one rejoices!* The neighbours have doubts and are divided (9:8–12). The religious leaders are divided and argue about tradition and miracles (9:13–17)! Fear and group pressure are brought to bear on the parents (9:18–23). Such extreme anger is engendered that the one healed is cast out (9:24–34)! What was the greatest day of his life may have turned out to be the worst because of the sick reactions of the healthy!

Christ's healing causes this double reaction. Those who know their need can be made whole and rejoice: those who pride themselves in their strength and normality frequently need to protect themselves by anger from having their weaknesses exposed.

John has Jesus sum up this phenomenon neatly when he says,

> It is for judgement that I have come into the world, so that those *without sight may see* and those *with sight turn blind*. (9:39)

Do not embark on healing ministry until you are prepared fully to face *both*. The light of God will enlighten those who welcome it, but blind those who fear it.

The shadow of the Cross touches all truly Christian healing ministry. Think of those who ministered Christ's healing in the New Testament . . . were not most of those that sprang to mind martyred?

When we ask questions about the appropriateness or suitability of having a healing service we are not asking questions at the same level as those about Harvest Suppers or rose bushes in the Memorial Garden!

Is the central core of the church open and ready for God's moving among them? Can they face the depth and disturbance of Christ's healing work? Healing is not like some spiritual 'soup' that the church need not itself taste but simply dole out to others! Healing is an open-ended invitation to God to come amongst us, to cleanse, remake, transform, set right, readjust, renew, change, – the list is endless!

Matthew gives a thumb-nail sketch of healing in ch. 21. It warrants study.

Jesus then went into the Temple and drove out all those who were selling and buying there; he upset the tables of the money changers and the chairs of those who were selling pigeons. 'According to scripture' he said 'my house will be called a house of prayer; but you are turning it into a robbers' den.' There were also blind and lame people who came to him in the Temple, and he cured them. At the sight of the wonderful things he did and of the children shouting, 'Hosanna to the Son of David' in the Temple, the chief priests and scribes were indignant. (12–15)

If Christ is invited to be present to heal, then he will not ignore our ecclesiastical and denominational sicknesses and focus just on those whom we tell him are in need! The Cleansing of the Temple provides us with a clear model of healing. The twin results of Christ's 'judgement' are again apparent. We must not let the indignation of the blinded eclipse the Hosannas of those whose eyes have been opened!

We cannot welcome the King unless we are willing to welcome his rule. The coming of the Christ results in the overthrow of Church-ianity. Those who have found their security in the *things* of Christ and not in Christ himself experience great trauma when their false religion is exposed.

If I seem not to be writing about healing services it is because it would not be kindness on my part simply to suggest that they are held on the basis of a few people wanting them, and not to warn you that unlike so much that goes on in church life, with a healing service one is stepping right into spiritual matters.

Some years ago Canon David Edwards bemoaned the Church's theological enthusiasms for 'the death of God, the suicide of the Church, the unknowability of Jesus, the impossibility of preaching and . . . the uncanny ability of so much contemporary church life to avoid mentioning matters such as God.' God forgive us; a number in our congregations have grown to know only a deceased God and a Church suicidal! Any experience of the living God and the Church *spiritual* is likely to come as a shock which they may – or may not – be able to take! It brings 'judgement'.

In relation to this judgement, it is very important not to lapse into what I call the stumbling-block-heresy. Some Christians take the inherent offence of the Cross (1 Cor. 1:23) to explain everyone else's negative reactions to their own thoughtless and insensitive behaviour!

All criticism, in whatever spirit it is given, should be taken and pondered carefully. God usually has much to teach us through our critics. We must avoid taking the 'judgement' too lightly or too heavily. It must not lead us to be over casual and careless on the one hand or hypersensitive and over-careful on the other. If we wait for the time when everyone is ready to welcome everything, then we shall wait for eternity. The knowledge that if we travel in a straight line we are bound to hit something sooner or later has helped me through a number of difficult patches!

Questions I would ask myself in a local situation would be:

(a) Does the congregation at large have a knowledge and balanced understanding of the Church's Ministry of Healing?

(b) Would such a step be at a tangent to the style

of our present church life or would it be a natural development of it?

(c) Does the subject arise out of a love for others and a real commitment to spiritual growth; or is it little more than a wish to leap on the latest bandwagon?

(d) Can they guess the cost, and are they willing to face it?

3. One Church or Ecumenical?

There is a time and a place for both. An ecumenical service is itself a healing experience and witness to the healing of the Church.

Quite often a local Council of Churches will consider holding such a service centrally, or one of the healing guilds will take the initiative. The Guild of Health in my own diocese (Guildford) holds an annual ecumenical healing service in the cathedral with twenty or more Christian priests and ministers laying on hands, and an invited speaker.

Sometimes a small joint effort brings the necessary encouragement for folk to start, on the two-heads-are-better-than-one principle.

The experience of many local churches is that their first healing service develops out of their own intercession group that meets to pray for the sick. Such groups are excellent and should be encouraged, but can sometimes result in the healing ministry appearing to be very fringe if their activity, time, place and numbers, relate in no way whatever to the ordinary Sunday congregation.

If public healing services are held by one church for itself, then the possibility of an ecumenical development at some later date ought to be kept in mind.

Some basic ecumenical groundwork could be done

by the lay-speakers of one parish visiting groups of another to share good grass-roots' experience.

There are no universal rules. In some situations the natural development will be within one local church, while in others the next step forward will be an ecumenical venture.

As any local church family open themselves to the work of the healing God in their midst, it will not be long before they become painfully aware of the *un*healed nature of our divided Church. Fortunately we do not have to wait for the Church to be healed before it can be an instrument of God's healing grace! But if we are not visibly healing our own ailments, why should others expect us to have any resources to heal theirs? We have been entrusted with the ministry of reconciliation (2 Cor. 5:18). Unreconciled Christians cannot fulfil it.

4. For the Church or Society?

Again there are no rigid rules.

There are certain things we need to note.

(i) There is always a danger that the Church's Healing Ministry is seen exclusively in terms of individual need. If 'holy huddles' have sapped the Church's mission-resources in the past, then there is a very great danger that 'holy *healing* huddles' will do so in the future.

'Healing', far from being the Church's ministry, can become the Church's *sickness* if it becomes preoccupied with self rather than service. To gaze at one's spiritual navel is not the goal of Christian healing!

(ii) It may well be right for services to take place among those and for those who are committed and taught *provided* such services are essentially regarded as equipment for the Church's task of mission. If, as William Temple is so frequently quoted as saying, 'The Church is the only society that exists for the benefit of its non-members', then whatever God gives by way of blessing is given not for its sitting but its sending!

'No U-Turn' is a good motto for the Church's Ministry of Healing and for public healing services. The *direction* of salvation/wholeness/healing is *outward*. A recurring theme in the healing stories of the New Testament is that of *going* rather than coming! '*Go* home to your people and tell them all that the Lord in his mercy has done for you' (Mark 5:19). The woman with the haemorrhage (Mark 5:34), Bartimaeus (Mark 10:52) and the leper (Mark 1:44) were each told to go.

It was only in *going* that the ten lepers were cured (Luke 17:19). Without going and obeying the blind man in John's gospel would have been doubly blind – with mud on his sightless eyes (9:7, see also Mark 2:12, 8:26, Luke 14:4)!

In one cathedral there was a regular intercession group which met, tucked away, in a side-chapel. The noise of the visitors was such that they asked for the use of a microphone and found themselves moved to a more exposed place. The visitors now witness the group's prayer and ministry through the Laying-on-of-hands. The occasion has moved – or been moved! – gently from in-reach to out-reach.

(iii) The place of a public healing service can only be assessed within the total life of a parish. It will be quite clear whether the local church offers merely an escape from society or a servicing point for it.

It is possible, as I have pointed out above when considering the 'Mature' stream of Christian healing (pp. 28–9), to be so over-careful about the healing ministry that it is virtually unknown to the faithful and society.

Although I am careful by nature, I have to admit that the New Testament witness seems to me to be considerably bolder than the Church's thinking at this present time. I predict that there will be a steady move away from filleted evangelism towards a fuller Gospel-evangelism that touches the whole person and his environment.

(iv) The Church cannot postpone its mission until it is whole and strong enough. That would postpone it indefinitely! Fortunately it is in our weakness that God's strength is perfected – so let's get on with it!

(v) The symbol of the Laying-on-of-hands is identical for commissioning and healing, and I do not think the two should be separated. Society should benefit from any good healing service – even if it is not 'open'.

5. *Eucharistic or not?*

The mainstream denominations are united in seeing that the *ideal* setting for the exercise of the Church's Ministry of Healing is the Eucharist. None, however, would confine such ministry to it.

An ecumenical occasion for a public healing service is not likely to be eucharistic, since our ecclesiastical sickness is such that the Lord's Supper is our place of greatest disunity.

If the event is geared to witness and outreach to which non-Christians are welcomed, then, again, a eucharistic setting would be likely to put at a distance those who matter most.

The advantages of a eucharistic setting are:

(i) It puts healing ministry at the heart of the gospel

declaration, and places it firmly in the context of salvation.

(ii) It puts what might be the unfamiliar with the security of the familiar. (I use 'security' here in no derogatory way. Folk will not easily accept new things if their context makes them feel uneasy.)

(iii) By having a strongly sacramental setting, it is likely to avoid the dangers of individualism and emotionalism.

(iv) The eucharistic congregation will be one which is known and most easily taught, prepared, and followed-up. It is likely to be a pastoral unit with its own resources for support.

There are certain difficulties as well.

(i) A usual Communion Service is, in most traditions, already something of an over-full service with a tight schedule. Folk do not take easily to the dropping of familiar items in order to include unfamiliar ones!

(ii) It is not likely to be suitable for an ecumenical or 'open' occasion.

If the service is the Eucharist, then it is likely that a decision will need to be taken about where the Laying-on-of-hands would come within it. There are two main positions, and each expresses something valid.

One view links it with confession and absolution, so the ministry is an extension or deepening of what is already the great healing act. It is then a restoration preparatory to personal Communion.

The other view (the one I favour) is to place the ministry after Communion has been received. Here it expresses a personal and deeper outworking of the blessing given in Communion. Since our healing is not that we should be strengthened to come to God but to be sent out by him, this placing encourages the necessary *outward* direction. If the Laying-on-of-hands is seen as essentially an individual blessing (see above pp. 72ff.), when it is placed towards the end of a service it becomes the final corporate blessing *expressed individually for those who wish*. Its innovation at this later position in the service is certainly the easiest development of what already is familiar. (In the event of all receiving God's blessing *individually*, the final corporate blessing should, of course, be omitted.)

There are some who quibble that 'nothing further need or can be given' after God's gift of the Holy Communion. If such critics accept the appropriateness of the customary corporate blessing they can have no theological grounds for objecting to it being given normally, i.e. individually.

A number of churches have Laying-on-of-hands and Anointing for those who wish at every Sunday Eucharist. When done so regularly the numbers are not great and the time of the service is not unduly prolonged. This has much to commend it. It places the healing ministry at the centre, and safeguards against any over-emphasis on healing services.

The most natural way, in many churches, for this to become the norm is to build upon the practice of blessing the non-communicants formally and semi-formally. It is then a small step to pray occasionally for communicants.

6. Once-off – or Regular?

If such ministry is being introduced, then, in those Christian streams that keep Saints' Days, St Luke's-tide provides an ideal occasion to focus on healing – and in a way which affirms God's working in medicine.

If once-off, those who are not in favour can escape the issues involved by not turning up, and then (not having witnessed a good healing service at first hand) say how heretical and emotional such things are! On the occasions when I have been asked to address an inaugural healing service I have often suggested that before anything is decided I visit the church council and spend the evening considering the Church's Ministry of Healing together. Once this is done, if the council decides on the 'go-ahead', any major split over the matter is avoided.

Each local situation is different, and God's will for it is different. In thinking through the alternatives my hope is that we might be alerted to hear from him what otherwise we might have missed because it was not part of our thinking.

9

Planning

If public healing services are times when we hope for people to encounter the healing love of God then we must be aware that much of that healing love should be experienced in *the quality of their encounter* with those around and the setting.

If folk are anxious because the service runs late and their return will create tension with the baby-sitter; if they have had a hassle parking their car and are embarrassed at arriving late; if they needed a toilet at the beginning of the service but none was available and they are in physical discomfort; if people around them are insensitive in their devotions; if they are confused about which book to use; if they feel guilty about their ignorance and inability about joining in strange responses and/or unfamiliar songs; if they are continually left in the dark about what will happen next; if they were not welcomed and made to feel at home . . . the list could be endless.

If those attending endure such things then the service may as well be cancelled, for by our failure really to love those who attend, we have in large measure denied them the experience of God's love in welcoming and accepting them.

These are central and *spiritual* matters! Those of us who believe in miracles and in God's intervention can sometimes lapse in what God demands of us and through us. I have attended a mid-winter service in which too much was 'left to the Spirit', and the Spirit had forgotten to turn on the heating!

Every Christian present is called to 'minister' God's love, not just those termed 'ministers'. There is just as much 'ministry' going on – or not going on – in the car park, at the toilets, at the door, with the books, and in the kitchen as there is at the altar rail.

If visitors experience the Church's love at the east end of the building and its indifference at the west end then there is much lacking in our concept of the Church's Ministry of Healing! I call for an improvement in east-west relationships!

Rather than describe the planning necessary for ecumenical and local, and for both 'closed' and 'open' services, I shall outline the planning for the larger event and leave the reader to reduce it accordingly for smaller situations. What follows is a fairly comprehensive check-list.

1. Spiritual Preparation

Regular and committed prayer for the occasion is top priority. As well as the obvious topics the following ought not to be overlooked.

(a) Prayer that those attending will be *only* those of God's choosing. (This rightly implies God's action to keep away those who would not at that particular moment benefit from attending, or who would cause any wrong disturbance, etc.)

(b) Prayer that God will prepare those whom he is gathering so that the service will play its rightful place in God's ongoing programme for their lives.

(c) Prayer for the place in which the service is to be held, that the Spirit of Christ would be present to

113

the exclusion of all that might disturb or that does not acknowledge Jesus as Lord.

(d) Prayer for the follow-up that the relevant caring communities may be sensitive to God's leading and be instruments of his care and support.

Other prayer topics are too obvious to mention!

At a conference I led in Holland arrangements were made for the chapel on the site to have Christians at prayer in it literally around the clock. Where there is such spiritual commitment the event will be a healing one whether the visiting speaker turns up or not! Parishes that lead the way will have whole nights of prayer. Regular fasting for such occasions is practised by many.

These details are not to discourage the small hesitant group, but to provide something of a goal at which to aim. God always 'means business', and it seems to be a law of spiritual life that there are particular blessings sooner or later when we 'mean business' as well. Such spiritual efforts are not, as might appear, Christian magic to bend God to our will, but expressions of the commitment and willingness for our wills to be realigned with his.

2. Speaker

I mention this second not because he or she is more important than all that follows, but because if it is planned to have a 'name', then the person is likely to require eighteen months' notice. The choice must reflect the view of the planning group. If the concept of the ministry is that it is essentially corporate, then care might need to be taken with certain individuals who would regard the occasion as their own to do exactly what they want with!

A few well-known speakers run roughshod over

their hosts' plans by talking infinitely longer than scheduled and then – to add insult to injury! – taking over ministry not allocated to them. That God blesses such occasions says more about God's grace than it does about the rightness of the speaker's failure to submit to his hosts and show elementary courtesy toward them.

The outside speaker (if one is planned) should primarily be the servant and the spokesman of the local leadership. Often the choice of name comes before the choice of subject or style of ministry. This is usually the wrong way round. It is better that the local leaders have a clear idea of the ministry and teaching required and *then* to ask for the one best able to fulfil it.

I have had many invitations which have encouraged me to do whatever I wanted and speak about anything I liked. This imposes an enormous spiritual burden on the speaker and usually means that he is being 'used' by his hosts to do all their praying, thinking, discerning and planning for them! No way!!

'Feel free to do whatever the Spirit leads you to do!' is at best an indication of trust, but at worst it can mean that no attempt has been made locally to discern what the Spirit wants, and that the outside speaker is being imported as a labour-saving device!

It is good, though diaries rarely allow it, if the outside speaker can make a preliminary visit and sit in on the planning committee/council of those arranging such an event.

3. *Date*

If a 'name' is wanted a priority list of three or four is a good idea. Some take months to reply. If the first two are unable to come, six months can easily be lost before the speaker is even known!

An ecumenical event can hardly be scheduled earlier than a year ahead, and will probably not fall on a Sunday. The cancelling of all evening services is sometimes done. Some are unwilling to do this because of the loss of income from their evening offertory. This can easily be overcome if in the planning the likely income of the churches is known in advance and the collection divided appropriately.

Unfortunately the Week of Prayer for Christian Unity is planned when evenings are dark, but it might provide an occasion for corporate as well as personal healing. Those who minister the Laying-on-of-hands first lay hands on each other. This could have particular meaning if preceded by, say, a litany of penitence.

St Luke's-tide I have already mentioned. Speakers who are known to talk on healing are in much demand at that time since so many healing groups and guilds have their annual events then.

Anglicans have, in addition, the Eighth Sunday before Easter on the theme 'Christ the Healer', and at least half a dozen Sundays with 'healing' Gospel readings.

4. Time

Those attending 'healing' events almost invariably number more than expected. (Just as conferences with 'healing' in their theme are usually fully booked!) Unless there has been exceptionally good planning the event is, therefore, likely to run late! It is wise to assume that it will take longer than planned, in which case an earlier rather than later start should be made.

Sometimes a preparatory meeting for prayer or meditation is arranged for a half an hour or more beforehand. This should not delay the start of the service.

5. Venue

The place of meeting will be dictated to by the *aim* of the meeting. If it is seen primarily as evangelism with healing accompaniment, then a non-church building may well be best. If it is seen primarily as Christian worship then a church is likely to be more appropriate.

In view of the importance of caring for those attending and thus expressing God's love in practical ways, the quality and facilities of the plant are important.

Does it have side room(s) for counselling? Has it facilities for wheelchairs? Has it accessible toilets? Adequate car parking? Is it on a bus route? Are the main pews open-ended or will those not at the centre be trapped against a wall (and thus find it difficult to come forward for the Laying-on-of-hands if most of their row remain seated)? Is the building a fairly quiet one for people to move around in? Is it attractive and welcoming? Does it speak of life or death? Is its arrangement an aid to what is planned? Is its amplification system adequate? Is it felt to be a place of prayer? Does it so strongly reflect one Christian tradition, either by its barrenness or clutter, that Christians of other streams would not quickly feel at ease in it?

6. Teaching

If the service has to be planned well ahead it is an ideal opportunity for the churches involved to set aside some time, e.g. Lent, or an autumn course, to study the subject of healing. The earlier chapters of this book might be used for that purpose, or other publications, e.g. the United Reformed Church's *Health and Healing* study kit (used by all denominations) or the report *The Church's Healing Ministry* (above pp. 19–25).

7. Publicity

The denominations are unanimous in their respective reports that considerable care be given to this. The usual advice is for mention to be made within church publications and circles rather than any mass publicity. If it is advertised at all widely then non-Christians of different faiths and of none may be expected to be present and the teaching of the service will have to include introductory material that in church circles would probably not have to be given (see chapter 11).

If it is planned as an outreach then the publicity should be wider, but those welcomed from outside ought not, I think, once in, to have to foot the bill for their invitation by being expected to donate to the collection! It can be stated that the collection is primarily for the regular worshippers and that newcomers are not expected to contribute. Such is the image of the Church that some 'raising' ministry might then be necessary for those who die of shock!

8. Service Leadership

Arrangements should be made well in advance for the Laying-on-of-hands to be administered, ideally, in pairs. Reserve teams should be on call to assist if the presiding minister so indicates. (This might be because the service is running late, or there seems to be a special pastoral situation that requires it.)

It is a mistake, on a large occasion, for the principal minister himself to be involved in the Laying-on-of-hands. At such services someone needs to *preside*. I have seen services run very late indeed because every available minister has become engaged in the Laying-on-of-hands, and everything has been endlessly held up because no one else felt themselves in the position to take the service on! (If the ministry of individual blessing seems likely to run the service late, let it go on during some/all of the remaining part of the service. It is not ideal, but it is better than endlessly detaining an entire congregation. It is no great distraction on a large occasion to be prayed over while a congregation is worshipping or singing.)

The president should orchestrate the event and *all involved should willingly come under his presidency* – and that includes the music department!

On countless occasions that I have attended, the worshippers have been made to endure every rehearsed item imposed as of *right*! All those taking part should be told clearly, well before the service, to be prepared to *contribute* certain items – but the president must be free to adjust and readjust the timings if the service is to be a good one.

If the speaker runs over, axe some verses of a hymn! If a testimony is given and takes twice the anticipated time (they usually do!) then drop a music item. If the crowd is double that which was anticipated, use your shorter stand-by Scripture reading(s), and axe a hymn. If the Laying-on-of-hands gets too prolonged then unscheduled but prepared music or singing might be introduced.

Presiding at such services, if they are to have both

the benefit of structure and the liberty of the Spirit (as should all worship!), is like dealing with a string of elastic bands between two fixed points! If one becomes overstretched another must be reduced! I know from my experience at Fountain Trust that it is quite possible to conclude gatherings of thousands – in which considerable freedom has been exercised – right on schedule! This, of course, requires a real team working together, all being willing to submit and each being willing to forego, if necessary, their planned contribution.

Such presiding can create ill feeling and personal hurt if it is not talked over and established from the word 'go' with all concerned. It is not easy, it requires discipline and sacrifice. I recall once having the time allocated for my carefully prepared talk halved at a moment's notice! I'm no saint! I didn't find it easy, but it was certainly right.

9. Service Staffing

The 'edges' of such services are important pastoral areas. There is often the odd person (and they may be very 'odd' indeed!) who lingers at the door, and others who clearly want to hover at the back. They are attracted yet fearful. It needs very, very sensitive caring if these 'smoking flaxes' are not to be quenched. How often I grieve when, on the platform, I see those with welcoming ministries desert their posts at the doors during the first hymn and take a cosy seat near the front for shelter! The fringes of gatherings should always be discreetly staffed by some of the most experienced and mature Christians. They should remain there throughout, to welcome late-comers, handle noisy doors, dispel the embarrassment of those who need toilets or have to leave early, answer questions of the inquisitive, and so on. The crowds in the pews do not need extra pastoral care, they are getting plenty in worship and ministry. Time and care should be unostentatiously lavished on fringers. On our care may depend their entry into the Kingdom of God. How many stories of changed lives – and sometimes famous ministries – have begun with folk being led (by what or whom they know not) to the fringe of a Christian gathering.

Counsellors not involved in laying on hands should be available, for there may be one or two for whom counselling is necessary and the altar rail is not the place to do it.

10. Printing

Three things in particular are useful.
(a) A service sheet, which, if not in full, gives folk a very clear idea of what is going to happen, together with details of when to stand and sit. Many are petrified of standing up or sitting down in the wrong place.
(b) Comments, thoughts and prayers for individual use before/after receiving the Laying-on-of-hands.
(c) A card for strangers to fill in to facilitate making contact and assist in follow-up. This might include name, address, phone number and boxes to tick if personally prayed for and/or would like a visit, magazine, etc. It is possible for (a), (b) and even (c) to be combined.

11. Other Practical Points

The usual common-sense steps taken for ordinary services apply no less to a public healing service, and hardly need mention, e.g. baby-sitting arrangements to enable couples to attend together; transport

for the elderly; possible light refreshments afterwards – a very useful way of initiating follow-up;
the roping-off of a rear section of chairs until the
beginning of the service so that late-comers may
have easily accessible seats (for the benefit of all
concerned). Tapes or a video might be made of the
talk given for use by church members and ministers
in the homes of the house-bound.

Some readers will be asking, 'But where is God
in all this?' Such a question contains its answer '*in
all this*'! Preparing is a difficult but worthwhile task.
Spiritually it is a John-the-Baptist ministry. Our
temporary preoccupation with practical things is
simply preparing a way for the coming of the Lord
and making his path straight. It is his coming for
which we work and which we await. We owe such
care both to the One who comes and to those who,
at our invitation, will await him.

10

Servicing

Services are aptly named for although it is not their aim, they are in fact our *servicing*. 'Forgive us all that is past and grant that we may serve you in *newness of life*' as an Anglican prayer of confession puts it.

Our servicing is a complex business, and, if we use the car analogy, we are all different models!

It is the *service* that services, not just isolated parts, like the Laying-on-of-hands that some may term 'ministry'.

God ministers to those present through the welcome, the atmosphere, the fellowship, the Scriptures, the teaching, the confession and absolution, the prayer, the testimony, the preaching, the praise, and so on.

Once we share that belief, then every item is of equal importance.

The service must be planned with great care, and the nature of worship understood.

Committee-liturgy, a hotchpotch of everyone's favourite item, should be avoided at all costs! An ecumenical committee may construct liturgy on the basis of fair representation! This too should be avoided. A good ecumenical service is simply a good service arranged ecumenically!

I have never had ice-cream with my soup, and that is not really surprising because it goes against the *natural order* of a meal. I have on many occasions suffered the liturgical equivalent when worship has been planned by those who do not understand it. My most recent experience was to have soup on my ice-cream(!) with a final hymn of the 'O come . . .' variety, inviting me to worship!

It is perfectly all right for worshippers not to understand worship, for, like cycling, it is meant to be done and enjoyed rather than analysed. But the planning of worship *must* be in the hands of those who not only do it, but understand it. Here, by way either of reminder or introduction, are some notes on the natural form of worship.

Public Worship

Consider this conversation:

'Hi son! I was hoping to meet you.'

'Hello Dad. I was hoping to see you too. I'm sorry I was late last night but I forgot . . .'

'That's all right, son, but I was concerned. Thank you for telling me.'

'Dad, could you lend me a fiver?'

'What for?'

'I want to get John a get-well present.'

'Yes, that's fine. Here you are. I was actually on my way to visit him now . . .'

'May I come with you?'

'Yes, delighted! I'll give you a lift . . .'

'Thanks, that's great!'

Such a conversation is *natural* and therefore has an ordered progression to it. It develops and advances a series of *responses*. The conversation includes recognition; greeting; apology; reconciliation; request; fresh response; redirection; fellowship, and joint action.

124

Worship is simply an organized meeting of this sort arranged for a crowd to meet with God.

Good worship is natural: poor worship is unnatural. Poor worship has no inner dynamic, and mere liveliness is no substitute. Good worship has a natural dynamic like the conversation above, and its various responses are very similar, in spite of their different names – 'adoration', 'confession', 'absolution', 'intercession', etc.

Good worship is a dynamic and developing two-way conversation between God and us, each side using *words*, *things*, *actions* and *silence*.

(a) WORDS

God speaks *to us* particularly by Scripture, teaching, testimony, prophecy, exhortation, absolution, commissioning, and blessing; also in certain 'manward' hymns, etc. e.g. 'There is a green hill . . .'

We speak *to God* in hymns, psalms, songs, and prayers containing our adoration, repentance, intercessions, thanksgiving and praise.

(b) THINGS

God particularly uses water, bread, wine, hands, oil, and certain other symbols, e.g. crib and cross.

We use our voices, hands, bodies, bread, wine, money (and, annually, tokens of harvest) when sharing with God.

(c) ACTIONS

God's manward actions include washing, breaking, outpouring, feeding, touching and anointing.

Our actions Godward are what we do with our *bodies*! Only a few are common to all Christian traditions: singing, speaking, standing – and, probably, donating! Others include kneeling, bowing, prostrating; hands together, clapping, hand-raising;

turning, walking, dancing; and making music. (Those who hold a negative, rather than healthy doctrine of Creation tend not to use their bodies. The so-called 'non-Conformist squat' coupled with a heavy frown and a pinched nose which many 'Bible-Christians' adopt for prayer falls far short of being Biblical!)

The naturalness of worship can be checked by asking of each item whether it is an appropriate response (manward or Godward) to the last. (The notices are usually awkward to place precisely because they form no natural place in the God-man man-God dialogue, their 'direction' being man-to-man, and 'horizontal'.)

It is better to grasp the natural structure of worship and for local Christians to work for something appropriate than to import, in detail, the services of others.

Each part of the service should be as clear as possible and taken at the tempo which will effectively 'minister' its contents to those present.

Particular attention ought to be paid to the penitential part, for the majority present, regular Christian worshippers included, will be riddled with guilt, and the healing nature of sins forgiven cannot be over-emphasized.

It is not always necessary to have a 'healing story' for the Scripture reading. Those attending will expect to encounter God. There are many readings that minister widely by declaring God's love and faithfulness.

A list of frequently chosen readings is given below.

Before we turn to personal ministry, mention must be made of the introduction. It is important to set people *at ease*, and this should be given by the adult who can best do it rather than automatically the host.

At an ecumenical service, the introduction might go something like this:

'We extend a very warm welcome to you all. We welcome friends from church A, B, and C. Some of you will have come in a group; some by yourselves. Just turn to your neighbour and find out their name and where they have come from . . .

'You have service sheets and these will enable you to relax and know what's coming next! Worship in the style that is natural for you. If you want to kneel, kneel; if you want to stand and raise your hands, do so. Let's relax and allow others to relax. Our unity is expressed by our being *together*, not by worshipping in any way that is unnatural to us.

'There are a number of stewards – you'll spot the discs they are wearing. Just signal to one if you want anything. Those who would find coming forward for prayer physically difficult and would like the ministers to pray for them in their seats, just raise a hand when the time comes.

'We will finish the service no later than X o'clock. If you have to leave earlier because of buses or babysitters just slip out whenever you need to.

'Some may not be able to sit for too long a period. There's no point in attending a 'healing' service and feeling worse after than you did before! If you would like ministers to pray with you during the first half hour then just indicate to your nearest steward, and we'll arrange that quite easily.

'If you are not a regular member of a local church and have just dropped in – a *special* welcome. We are particularly glad to meet new friends, and to help us keep in touch there is a card in your place.

If you could fill it in during refreshments afterwards it would help us keep in touch with you.'

The primary task of such an introduction is not the imparting of vital information at all! It is an immediate statement to every single individual present, 'We're God's people and we love you as he does. You matter greatly to us, you are our care and concern. We accept you and welcome you.'

We naturally treat well those whom we love, and casually those who mean nothing to us.

Such love goes a long way to driving out the fear which all of us experience in unfamiliar surroundings and which creates '*dis-ease*'. It is worth noting that the opposite of 'dis-ease' and 'un-ease' is *ease*. We cannot be natural if we are un-easy, and as Bishop Michael Marshall points out in his excellent book *Renewal in Worship*, the first requirement for the supernatural is to be natural!

(It is no accident that many religious cults – and businesses – foster techniques of warmth and welcome to enslave others.) In contrast we care, simply because we care. We have no strings attached or ulterior aim.

One of the main difficulties in a public healing service is the *time* it takes to pray and lay on hands if the number coming forward is great. Such ministry to individuals needs to be short, but neither hurried nor skimped, otherwise we are felt to minister God's rejection rather than his love!

If organizers assume that the congregation will be *double* their expectations and that all will come forward their planning will probably be right!

A considerable number of teams ready to lay on hands, including a number of reserve teams, is essential.

The Laying-on-of-hands need not be confined to

the Communion rail, but can also be administered at other 'stations' around the building. In extremely busy and crowded conditions folk may just queue and receive their prayer and blessing standing.

At any one time during this ministry perhaps nine-tenths of the congregation are sitting with nothing to do. It will always include those who feel guilty and uneasy at having missed the opportunity to come forward. I have, on occasions, gone down into the centre of the nave while Laying-on-of-hands ministry has been going on, and spoken to the remainder. I have tried to assure them that what they see at a distance are visible symbols of God being present and ministering among us, that he is no more busy at the East End than he is *here* (i.e. within the seated congregation), and to use this time to thank him for his presence; to share with him their areas of anxiety; and ask God to touch them with his healing hand. I have sometimes led a general prayer for those who have not gone forward. It is important to try and minimize the impression that God is wonderfully busy *elsewhere* in the building. One criticism of John Wimber's style would be that when in an enormous crowd he indicates what God is actively doing in some part of it, this prompts folk to focus elsewhere rather than it being taken as an assurance of his presence *with me here*.

So many feel perpetually condemned that if they fail to come forward it will reinforce their own negative image – 'of course, it was all right for *them*!'

Jesus, as I have noted above (pp. 61–2), at the healing Pool of Bethesda, left those who could avail themselves of God's healing and gave his attention to the one who for personal reasons kept missing the opportunity (John 5:1–15).

At services that purport to be 'healing' ones we

ought to be particularly sensitive to those who, for whatever reasons, find themselves somewhat cut off or on the fringe of what is happening.

My suggestion that each person present greets his or her neighbour during the introduction is mainly to ensure that early on the 'fringe' members have the experience of being affirmed and noticed. (Much of Christ's healing ministry stemmed from his first stopping and, as Doctor Luke in particular stresses, *seeing* (7:13, 13:12, 17:14).)

Orders of service are printed in many books, among them the Baptist *Services of Healing*, the United Reformed *Healing Services* (from their study kit), the Methodist *Healing is Wholeness* by Howard Booth, and John Gunstone's *The Lord is our Healer*. There is little to choose between them, but here reproduced from page 190 is Canon Gunstone's model.

Introduction
    Hymn
    Notices
    Preparatory prayer
Ministry of the Word of God
    Scripture reading
    Hymn, psalm, canticle or song
    Scripture reading
    Sermon and/or testimony
Ministry of Prayer for Healing
    General confession and absolution
    Affirmation of faith
    Intercessions
    Laying on of hands (and anointing)
    Act of prayer and thanksgiving
    Dismissal

I would strongly advocate the use of the Lord's

Prayer in the first section, since informal or extempore prayer almost invariably omits both forgiveness and protection from evil – two important elements in healing!

As listed it appears that John Gunstone is thinking of the sermon and a testimony as alternatives. His own comments clearly indicate that the testimony should enhance the sermon, not replace it. I would, personally, insist on the exposition of Scripture.

The intercessions should not exclusively be concerned with the needs of those present, but be healthily aware of the needs of others.

Those of the charismatic stream who have experienced Christ's healing within charismatic-style worship tend to equate the two and assume that anything that is 'really of the Spirit' must be charismatic in style.

The issue is a sensitive one because people's feelings are involved. The criterion is what is appropriate.

A ruthless scrapping of what is familiar to impose what is not, increases unease rather than healing. Our Lord ministered sensitively to people where and as they were, he did not foist on them requirements of religious behaviour or belief. If Christ generously healed last week to the accompaniment of a guitar he will not go off in a huff if this week our care and sensitivity have led us to use the organ! I dislike writing in that way, but my experience tells me that our enthusiasm can so often lead to our making God ridiculously smaller rather than wonderfully greater.

There are, indeed, abundant blessings to be had in charismatic styles of worship with their greater liberty and warmth, but charismatics must not assume that healing services require expressions of charismatic spirituality to function well. On the other hand, those not in the charismatic tradition should not be shut to the leading of the Spirit into rich but unfamiliar things.

The right thing at the wrong time is *wrong*. Like all pastoral activities, a loving sensitivity is required.

If such services are to minister the riches of God it is important that they are not put into some party's straight-jacket! I recall attending a packed service in a vast church. The final rousing hymn should have shaken the neighbourhood, but it faltered disastrously. The powers-that-be, knowing the event was 'charismatic', had locked up the organ-case (and organist as well for all I know!), and a lone guitarist tried valiantly but in vain to do the impossible!

I have dealt with the planning of the service. In the following chapter I shall deal with the teaching and the ministering contained in it.

By way of an appendix to this chapter, here is a list of some suitable Bible readings. I do not know who first compiled it, but it is reprinted in the Methodist *Services of Healing*, the Baptist *Services of Healing*, and the United Reformed Church's *Healing Services*. With such weighty authority behind it, need I say more, except to indicate briefly what each passage is about.

Isaiah 40:1–11 (Comfort my people)
    53:4–12 (By his stripes we are healed)
    54:7–10 (Compassion with everlasting love)
    58:1,6 and 9 (Transgression, deliverance, answer)
Matthew 5:1–12 (Beatitudes)
    6:25–34 (Heavenly Father cares for you)
Mark 1:21–34 (Exorcism and evening healings)
    *2:1–12 (Paralytic carried by friends)
    9:14–29 (The father with the epileptic demoniac)

Luke 7:18–29 (Blind see! Lame walk! Lepers are cleansed!)

9:1–6 (Commissioning of the Twelve)

10:1–9 and 38–42 (The Seventy plus Martha and Mary)

11:5–13 (Heavenly Father gives good things)

John 9 (Blind man healed plus negative reactions!)

14:12–17 (Ask anything in my name. The Comforter)

Acts 3:1–16 (Peter and John heal the cripple)

28:7–10 (Healing of Publius and the sick at Malta)

*2 Corinthians 12:7–10 (God's strength perfected in weakness)

*James 5:13–16 (Christian sick anointed by elders)

(The passages marked with * are the readings of the Anglican lectionary for the theme of Christ the Healer.)

The Baptist publication includes nineteen other Old Testament readings including readings on reconciliation (Gen. 45:1–28), forgiveness (1 Sam. 16:14ff), and caring (2 Sam. 9:1–13).

Among the Psalms commended are 23, 27, 30, 34, 43, 46, 51, 86, 91, 103, 116, 121, 139, and 143 (omitting v. 12).

A surprising omission from the list of Scripture readings is Luke 4:14–21, Christ's manifesto 'The Spirit of the Lord is upon me', ending, 'Today has this Scripture been fulfilled in your hearing.'

Twenty-four prayers each based on a passage of Scripture will be found in my pamphlet *Twenty-Four Healing Prayers*, and I commend warmly John Gunstone's book *Prayers for Healing*.

It goes without saying that Scripture reading should always be done by those best able to do it. Scripture is itself a minister of healing. It is sharper than any two-edged sword. Do not put it in the hands of those whose style will blunt it or render it ineffective, nor those who would use it to sharpen their own image!

A solo song would not be allocated to an ecumenical representative – why should a solo reading?

11

Teaching

When the public healing service is widely known and attended by non-Christians and the uninstructed it is important that right teaching be given. The task is, I think, a difficult one. The faithful will not need to hear what has to be said to the pagans, and will rightly expect to be 'fed' by the word given.

One solution is for an explanation of the service to be given as part of the introduction (or soon after). The other solution is for the speaker to gear his message to both believers and non-believers.

Some years ago, on the fortieth anniversary of VE Day to be precise, I was speaking at the Guild of Health's annual healing service in Guildford Cathedral.

Prior to the service I had prepared and printed my text in full, and given a copy to the presiding minister for his veto and to help him 'marry' the different elements of the service. (My printed copies I made available after the service, since this encourages the evening's ministry to be taken up again in homes, prayer groups and Bible groups.)

At the service itself the presiding minister omitted most of his usual introduction, which surprised me. Afterwards I learned from him that he felt that my sermon had included the basic introductory teaching that visitors needed.

It is printed in full below as an example of one

way in which this difficulty may be tackled. It is also as concise an expression of the points of this chapter as I am able to make!

There was one earlier reading from Luke 8:40–8.

I would not describe this evening as a 'healing service' but as a '*Christian* healing service', and there is an important difference. There are a multitude of ways in which men and women may gather to tap the healing forces of the natural and the supernatural. Some might seek the healing by the touch of another – rather as a run-down car battery can get a temporary boost by jump-leads to another.

Others would seek healing, reasonably enough, by the touch of a healer. With the large number of ministers who will pray with the Laying-on-of-hands, such an approach leads to great emphasis on the minister and the feeling that it is vital to get the best one to ensure results!

Some here will be hoping to be freed from some physical malady, and hope there will be some magical cure.

That's all right, perhaps, for 'healing'. But '*Christian healing*' is rather different. This very building is planned as a cross, and Christian healing is essentially *coming to Christ*; to a Christ who was not blessed by a painless and long life, but a Christ who experienced an untimely and excruciating death on a cross.

He died that we might be forgiven,
he died to make us good;
that we might go at last to heaven
saved by his precious blood.

This seems a long way from the migraine, or the arthritis, or the burden you carry tonight.

Truly *Christian healing* is nearly mind-blowing! If 'healing' is likened to a black and white snap, 'Christian healing' is a three-dimensional, high fidelity, glorious Technicolor wider-screen epic! Christian healing shatters all records and barriers. It explodes our thinking about healing. Christian healing touches not just your body – but you! Christian healing touches not just the next ten or twenty years – but *eternity*! Christian healing is not securing long life, but a foretaste of everlasting life! Christian healing is not about postponing or avoiding death, but about victory over it! God's offer of the gospel means to those who accept it a far greater 've' – VICTORY FOR EVERYONE!

Christian healing is not the ministry of some healer, with the shadowy figure of Christ somewhere in the background. It is the ministry of the Risen Christ himself who promises that when two or three are gathered together in his name that he will be in their midst (Matt. 18:20).

This makes a great difference to our thinking about this service and our expectations.

If we believe that Christ is distant, then we will be tempted to attach enormous importance to anyone with a 'hot line' to him. If Christ is absent, then ministers will be seen as the sole 'channels' of his healing power. Indeed they are channels, but such concepts are far too small, far too trivial to reflect the exciting truth – the LORD IS HERE! HIS SPIRIT IS WITH US! With us and present to touch, to convict and to forgive, to heal, to encourage, to bless, to guide, to renew and to transform.

If we have an inadequate view of an occasion like this it can lead to great anxiety and disappointment. Those who know themselves to have been too slow or too shy to go forward to be prayed over, spend the time of public ministry assuming that Jesus is busy up the front, and they miss his presence, care, and active healing love for them *where they are*. To be here at all is to be where the action is: because the Lord IS here; his Spirit IS with us. St Luke, the doctor, once used the phrase 'the power of the Lord was present to heal' (5:17). The Lord IS here!

The ministers do not act like so many spiritual hose-pipes bringing living water just to row one while leaving row thirty in drought! Ministers help express in word and deed in a few particular places with a few particular people what their Lord, Christ Jesus, is saying and doing as he ministers to all of us.

Christ's healing work will not delay until item nine on your sheets! It has already begun! It began in calling you to attend. Christ knows – and wishes us to know – that all our worship, our praise, our repentance, our prayers, our fellowship, and our openness to his Word in Scripture are all means by which he heals. They are means whereby we recover again that healed style of living, which he commanded us, loving God with all our heart and soul, mind and strength, and our neighbour as we love ourselves.

Our worship puts right all our priorities and relationships once again; our sins find forgiveness; our differences are reconciled; and God who is 'our health and salvation' is once more given priority over all else.

If a Christian healing service is essentially a *coming to Christ*, then it is a coming by us not to bully, or to bargain, but to submit.

Certain formal letters used to end with '*I am, my Lord, your obedient servant*.'

Neither Lordship nor obedience is very popular nowadays, but without them this service would be nothing. For in coming to Christ as 'LORD' it means that it is not we who try to exert power over him that he should comply to our will; but that he lavishes his power upon us to equip us to do his. Coming to the 'Lord' means that we do not tap some spiritual source, but offer ourselves to the Spirit of Jesus for his use in the world.

We come not to tell the Lord what he must do for his servant, but to listen, to learn, and to be equipped for what the servant must do for his Lord.

In our Gospel reading earlier (Luke 8:40–8) we heard of two events in the ministry of Jesus, events which show different ways of coming to the Lord.

The woman, you remember, suffering from constant haemorrhaging, comes not to meet Jesus face-to-face, but comes behind him to take a cure from him. She doesn't ask him, but avoids him. She hopes to remain anonymous; to shelter in the crowd. She hopes to grab what she can and slip away unnoticed!

I sympathize with her and understand her well. We are all shy, and hers was a very English trait to keep her religion to herself, and to avoid saying or doing anything noticeable in public.

She receives a physical cure, but it was something she took, not something she was given. It reflected her narrow preoccupation with herself, not the richness of Christ's loving concern for her as a whole person.

So Christ, although rushing to a dying teenager, STOPS! (I wonder what Jairus thought of that!) Christ then starts to make the cure blossom into a healing!

He first demands that she meet him face-to-face. This is just what she hoped to avoid, and it is initially very costly for her, for it means her being noticed, speaking in public and apologizing. (Three things that most of us dread!)

Christ loves her enough to be tough with her, knowing that he can minister real healing only when she is freed to have it on his terms rather than her own. So he continues the ministry which had begun by a physical healing, by healing next *her relationship to him* – 'My daughter'. To have lived with a physical cure but with an unhealed relationship with the Great Physician would not really have been a healing.

After healing the relationship, Christ heals *her wrong belief* by stressing that it was her faith-relationship to him that brought them together which had provided the basis for the cure – not some psychic energy flowing from his robes.

Healing can become a sickness when it gets too turned-in on itself; and the relationship between the sufferer and the healer can also become sick if it leads to what has been called a 'gruesome-twosome'! So Christ commands her to go as he did in so many of the Gospel healing stories, thus healing *the direction of her life*.

The woman began by trembling on the ground before Christ, fearful and guilty at her act of spiritual pick-pocketing. To have left his presence with her guilt remaining would have been to have had a cured body but a sick soul. Christ longed for her, as he longs for us, to receive his touch on our whole lives, body, mind, spirit, past, present, future, relationships, possessions, and so much more.

So to her guilt and fear the Lord Jesus Christ

ministers with the great Jewish word of blessing –
God's *peace*. Have so few words ever ministered
so much?

Daughter,
your faith has healed you,
go
in peace.

In these last words, Jesus adds the authority of
his word to her experience. Once established as
'Lord', he freely gives her what she had stolen
from him – and much more!

The woman, with whom so many of us can
identify, came as she could to Jesus. Jesus does
not judge her or condemn her. She experiences
enough shame without his adding to it!

He encourages her.

He addresses himself not just to the ailment,
but to her, the whole person. So his healing touch
is truly upon her – her body, her relationship with
him, her beliefs, the direction of her life, her fears
and her guilt; physical, spiritual, mental, social,
and inner healing.

The difference between a healing service and a
'*Christian healing* service' is that in a Christian
healing service we come not to steal a cure from
God, but we come afresh – or maybe for the first
time – *to Christ*. We come not behind his back,
but face-to-face, not trying to lord it over him
to get what we want, but allowing his love and
generosity to be LORD over us. We come for something which often includes physical cure, but is
far, far, far, far greater. We come for Jesus to
touch us, not just our ailments.

Jairus, in the story, was a leader of the Jewish
faith, and knew how to come to Jesus.

Jesus did not have to show him, for, as Mark

and Luke both tell us, he put pride aside, and *fell at Jesus' feet*.

The woman had brought her need to Jesus but held herself back from his fullest blessing.

Jairus swallows his pride, and comes humbly and *voluntarily* to the same position which the woman eventually reached in relation to Jesus – he came and *fell at his feet*.

It is at the feet of Jesus, the Christ, that *Christian healing* really starts. For when we kneel before him we are most conscious of our dependence on him, most conscious of his call that we should serve him; most conscious of what he is telling us; most willing to obey, and to receive from him that healing which is his equipment for us, as we go forth as soldiers and servants fighting under the banner of Christ against sin, the world, and the devil.

Thanks be to God who gives us the victory through our Lord Jesus Christ.

There are not many Scriptures that, to my mind, lend themselves quite so easily to this particular problem! Oddly, among many Christians, the action of the woman in touching Christ's garment is taken as a model for us. Line pictures of her doing so adorn a number of books on the healing ministry!

At the service at which the above was given the hymn 'The Healing God' was used, as printed below. This, not unlike the sermon, was designed as a teaching tool. It was written in an attempt to modify the two polarities about healing among Christians.

On the one hand it was written to correct those who assume that the gospel has nothing whatever to do with healing, and on the other to correct those who think that the only thing that really matters is physical cure!

Against the first view, the hymn piles up a great heap of healing-related themes linked to the persons and work of God in Trinity.

Against the second view, i.e. that physical cure is all that matters, is the fact that out of thirty-two lines, only half a line 'Cure of body' (v. 3) needs to be allocated to it!

It was written for the tune *Hyfrydol*, but it was sung to *Abbotts Leigh* – and sounded much better!

1. Healing God, Almighty Father,
   Active throughout history;
   Ever saving, guiding, working
   For Your children to be free.
   Shepherd, King, inspiring prophets
   To foresee Your suffering role –
   Lord, we raise our prayers and voices
   Make us one and make us whole.

2. Healing Christ, God's Word incarnate,
   Reconciling man to man.
   God's atonement, dying for us
   In His great redemptive plan.
   'Jesus', Saviour, Healer, Victor
   Drawing out for us death's sting.
   Lord, we bow our hearts in worship
   And united praises bring.

3. Healing Spirit, Christ-anointing
   Raising to new Life in him;
   Help to poor; release to captives;
   Cure of body; health within.
   Life-renewing and empowering
   Christ-like service to the lost.
   Lord, we pray 'Renew Your wonders
   As of a new Pentecost!'

4. Healing Church, called-out and chosen
   To enlarge God's Kingdom here,
   Lord-obeying; Spirit-strengthened
   To bring God's salvation near.
   For creation's reconciling
   Gifts of love in us release.
   Father, Son and Holy Spirit
   'Make us instruments of peace'.
   (From *Mission Praise 2*. (c) J. Richards)

The quotations from Pope John (v. 3), and St Francis (v. 4) add an ecumenical dimension. The charismatic movement may well have been born from the first, and the well-known prayer of St Francis has always been, to my mind, *the* great prayer of the Christian Healing Ministry.

I will end this chapter with it as a very suitable lead-in to the difficult and delicate subject of the next chapter – ministering the Laying-on-of-hands semi-formally, i.e. with extempore responses to spoken needs.

Lord, make me an instrument of your peace.
Where there is hatred, let me sow love;
where there is injury, pardon;
where there is discord, union;
where there is doubt, faith;
where there is despair, hope;
where there is darkness, light;
where there is sadness, joy;
for your mercy and truth's sake.
O Divine Master, grant that I may not so much seek
to be consoled as to console,
to be understood as to understand,
to be loved as to love,
for it is in giving that we receive,

it is in pardoning that we are pardoned,
it is in dying that we are born to eternal life.

(From *The Sunday Missal*)

12

Loving

In this chapter I shall write about ministering the
Laying-on-of-hands when done semi-formally, i.e.
praying *in response* to what the person has shared
with the ministers involved.

This is not *about* the Laying-on-of-hands and its
meaning, which I have already dealt with fully in
chapter 6. Here I shall focus exclusively on doing
the actual ministry. There is very little indeed
written about this, so I shall write in some detail.

I have tried in all earlier chapters to express the
mind of the Church on all the great healing themes
and practices. On this subject there is much Church
practice, but its mind has not yet been verbally
expressed or formulated. Perhaps it never will, for
it is the exercise of a spiritual art, not a spiritual
science.

I claim no expertise, but some experience. What
follows is something of an account of how I myself
'tick' when doing it. It has absolutely no formal
authority behind it whatsoever!

Pairs

As has already been stated this is desirable. It is less
necessary with formal Laying-on-of-hands in which
the ministers do not respond personally to needs
expressed. When semi-formal ministry is undertaken

– and this is probably the *usual* style in healing services – then the ministering partner is wellnigh indispensable.

Ideally the two ministers should work together on more than one occasion to build up a trust and rapport. From this can flow a quality of ministering that is genuinely exciting!

It is good if the pair have complementary gifts and insights, and a man and woman team is often good. Another useful mix is to have an experienced minister and one fairly new to this ministry working together so that the 'junior' can learn (almost unconsciously) by sharing.

It is particularly good to have Christians from the medical profession taking part in such teams.

The most often used arrangement is for each to take it in turn to lead the ministry with the then 'number two' supporting.

There are occasions when a nod, or knowing look from one minister will break the sequence, and the 'unscheduled' minister seems more appropriate.

If I am ministering with a woman-minister, and find my thoughts completely distracted by the blonde Swedish au pair kneeling before me, I will (I think wisely!) skip a turn rather than battle unsuccessfully with my enjoyable but inappropriate thoughts!

We have to be careful (in our culture) when touching others. We each have our own 'space bubble' around us, with very strict rules about who can invade it and how! This is right. Touching usually expresses intimacy, whether of parents and children or of those in love. Spiritual ministry of necessity also operates at a degree of intimacy that some people might not ever otherwise experience. When personal matters are shared with us, and when we touch those to whom we are ministering in Christ's name, we are on hallowed ground.

When ministering in pairs, if one gets tired and his concentration lapses, a nod to the other will forego the leadership sequence for a turn or two.

Most ministers will feel unsure at times. 'What will people think of me and my ministry if this person in a wheelchair isn't instantly cured!?' In this situation the minister with the greater experience might naturally move into the leadership role; not, I hasten to add, because he will bring a greater power of healing, but because the pain and the paradox of the Christian Healing Ministry will be something he has learnt to live with!

The verbal ministering need not be confined to the 'leader'. If the second minister discerns a Scripture that might be helpful to the sufferer (as distinct from one which is given for the ministers), he might share it briefly, or a quick word of counsel, or even a 'Can you see me afterwards?'

There are, in such circumstances, *two* two-way conversations going on at the same time. First, there is the person sharing verbally with the minister, to which the minister must listen and respond. Second, there is the inaudible two-way conversation going on between the one in need and God. The two may not always relate!

Most of us do not have that spiritual hot line to God so familiar to us from the autobiographies of those who publish accounts of their own ministries! Some leaders will, I am sure, find the two-way conversations easy. The rest of us, however, will be helped by ministering in pairs: the 'leader' fully active in expressing God's acceptance and love, in listening and responding, and the second minister detaching himself a little and seeking to discern the inaudible.

The person matters. Like Jesus we have initially to accept them as they are even if later we are privileged to lead them a step forward. If fear has caused a person to share the irrelevant, then we must begin with it. To switch off the person in order to listen to God sounds pious enough but is spiritually arrogant, theologically wrong and pastorally inappropriate! The spiritual recollection of the second minister may well enable the first to speak and act aright. If the team develops in mutual trust then the second minister may in time learn how rightly to enrich the ministry more directly by steering it to the point not discerned by the leader.

Channels?

I used to accept the usual concept that I was a 'channel' for God's love and words, but have since modified that. It implies that the needy person *only* experiences God through what I do or say. This concept places a quite enormous burden on any conscientious minister, for each word can become a matter of life or death!

The channel image always made me think of a house's fall-pipe (sometimes called 'drain-pipe'), at the top of which Almighty God was trying to pour down barrels of water, while I constituted its bottom end. Unfortunately, at the lower end, my sinfulness, disobedience, weakness and so on gummed up the pipe like an old bird's nest, letting only trickles of God's blessing reach their destination!

I do not reject such a concept, and I prepare for such ministry by deliberately tackling the bird's nest material in my life which might block God's grace.

My experience of, amongst other things, God present to heal without any visible 'channels' has convinced me that it is too narrow a concept. The outpouring of his blessing is never restricted to such channels, but generously overflows them.

This has, to me, made a very great difference to ministry of this kind. Instead of being in some sense the 'key' that makes the God-person encounter possible (or inhibits it), I now regard myself more as standing on the touch-line of an encounter which is already taking place.

I feel that my job in laying on hands and praying is not to direct the right amount of divine power in the right direction – like some spiritual laser! I believe instead that God and the needy person have already met; that there is a great healing encounter taking place, and that I am privileged to be in attendance.

Almost everything that is taking place is invisible and inaudible. My task is to try and make a little visible and a little audible something of what I think may be going on between God and the person concerned. I feel under a considerable responsibility to express this well, but I am no longer crushed by the burden that everything good will depend on my excellence!

I have not rejected the 'channel' concept but I no longer feel crushed by it. Speaking purely for myself, I think I now minister *better*. My earlier anxiety has been replaced by a greater relaxation, and my over-conscientiousness has given way to a greater liberty.

I was quite immeasurably helped by a comment of my dear friend Fr Jim McManus C SS R (author of *The Healing Power of the Sacraments*) when he said of healing ministry, 'If a person is cured I don't take the credit; if they're not – I don't take the blame!' It is so easy for the normal healthy neurotic like myself rightly to shun all the credit but wrongly to take all the blame!

Blessing on Behalf of Others

Virtually every public healing service will include those who come for Christ's touch not for themselves but for another. It may be for a relation or another member of the spiritual family. The issue has been debated in the church press, and it seems to be a deep and instinctive action of caring people. (I am sure I would do the same were a loved one of mine suffering.)

The late Revd George Bennett testified from his vast and world-wide experience that he had hardly had a service in which clergy or members of religious orders had not come forward for blessing by proxy. The practice is likely to be always with us.

Does Scripture give us any guidelines? There is no New Testament example of this particular use. There is, however, ample evidence of healing taking place at a distance which has in some sense been 'bridged' by a person or a thing coming between Christ and the sufferer (e.g. Mark 7:29–30, Luke 7:10, John 4:50, Mark 5:28, 6:56, Acts 5:15, 19:12). If a robe, a cloth, or a shadow even, can bring Christ's healing to the sick, one can hardly prevent (on Biblical grounds) a praying Christian who desires to do the same!

In situations where the Laying-on-of-hands is requested by proxy there are two people in need: the sick person and the individual who has come forward. This has always led me to pray first for the sufferer with the Laying-on-of-hands in proxy and then, quite separately – as if ministering to two people – for the person before me with the Laying-on-of-hands.

Sometimes the burdens carried by those alongside the ill are greater than the burden of actual sickness. God is generous. I am sure he does not want such people leaving without a renewed awareness that God is very specially with *them*, on whom they have been able to cast their burden because he cares for them (1 Pet. 5:7).

A surprising number of people who have the Laying-on-of-hands on behalf of another are themselves blessed or healed. (I suspect this is related to their freedom from self-preoccupation so that God's healing grace within them has less barriers to overcome than is usual with most of the rest of us!)

Other Double Ministries

A number of clergy in ordinary eucharistic settings administer Holy Communion to pregnant mothers and add a special blessing for the child by prayer with the Laying-on-of-hands on the mother.

With so many in society accepting the killing of the unborn as normal, Christians should not be reticent in promoting their blessing.

At public healing services it will often be noticed that husbands and wives join the queue for prayer. The closeness of some couples is sometimes clear. I have on occasions asked whether they would like to kneel together. A few times the invitation was declined, but more often the offer was appreciated. (It depends, of course, on the needs of each as to whether being together is appropriate.)

Counselling

Prayer and blessing must not be confused with counselling. It is not an impoverished version of counselling; it is a valid ministry in its own right.

To pray over people and give them God's blessing (whether formally or semi-formally) is as complete a ministry as administering Communion to them or reading them Scripture. If we do the latter without any unease that it is 'partial', we should lay on hands similarly.

If we are not convinced of this we will feel guilty that at a healing service, so little time can be allocated to any one individual.

(I have experienced healing services overrun by *hours* because the leaders concerned confused the ministry of semi-formal prayer with counselling.)

Many coming forward would benefit from counselling, but public ministry at a public service is the wrong place, although it may well provide the right beginning. Quite often a new grace will be given to enable real needs to be faced and to melt the pride that had made earlier help impossible.

Here are some points related to the counselling demand.

1. When the prayer and Laying-on-of-hands ministry is described at the service, what is expected can and should be outlined. For example, 'Those who want to be prayed over and to be individually blessed with the Laying-on-of-hands, go forward . . . You'll appreciate that this is not an opportunity for counselling, but if you have a topic for which you would particularly like prayer, do mention it briefly to the ministers.'

2. Those ministering will be helped by the conviction that our Lord knows all about the troubled situation,

and does not need to be told the sufferer's one-sided and partial version of it! Christ's healing touch does not depend on his first hearing the case history! Ministers will also be helped by the assurance that the healing event in which they are engaged is but one in a life-long programme that God is working out in the person's history. Our ministry will not set the sufferers free from life's problems, and even the most miraculous cure does not guarantee permanent health. (Even Lazarus died!)

We are not the Lord of the person's history; our ministry is just today's step. Many others will have been, and will be involved, past and present. We are one of a large team.

3. The limitations and opportunities of such ministry are shown by the following story. I recall, years ago, inviting a Pentecostalist minister to a small monthly service with the Laying-on-of-hands of my then parish intercession group. The numbers were small and I regularly prayed over them. I invited him, therefore, to lay on hands and to lead the ministry over each person.

On three occasions just before starting to pray over the next person, he paused, and addressed the previous one with the words 'I think maybe we ought to have a chat afterwards!' I knew the individuals well: how right he was!

One follow-up of that story is worth relating. I was present when he later saw each of them. To one he said, 'My poor dear, you've suffered an enormous personal loss, haven't you?' She immediately broke down and cried. She had. Her brother had died, and I, her parish priest, had never known of it for she kept her grief to herself!

The gifts of such spiritual insights have enriched the Church in every age, and have characterized the

ministries of so many of her pastors. Of the Curé
d'Ars it has been written, 'It quickly became
common knowledge that the Abbé Vianney could
read men's consciences and was reputed to work
miracles.'[1] More recently such 'charisms' have
graced the renewal or charism-atic movement, and
been equated with St Paul's 'gift of knowledge' (1
Cor. 12:8), although not traditionally so interpreted
by Protestant Christians. The terminology does not
concern me, but the need for spiritual sensitivity
does! Spiritual insight may well be founded upon
professional capabilities and natural gifts, but experience shows that it can, at times, be quite remarkably
different.

The Pentecostalist pastor may have discerned the
bereavement at the time of the Laying-on-of-hands.
If he did, he was wise and mature enough only to
use his insight at the right place. The public service
would not have been the *appropriate* place for the
surfacing of her grief.

Such gifts differ from psychic awareness which
may be a person's permanent ability in which the
unknown constantly intrudes for good or ill. A spiritual gift is given only when appropriate to make a
positive pastoral contribution. Our Lord had such
insight into the life of the Samaritan woman at the
well (John 4:18), and Peter knew the hearts of
Ananias and his wife (Acts 5:3ff).

Experiencing such a gift is a very mixed blessing!
With it comes the responsibility of knowing when,
where, and how to use it. I expect I lack the maturity
to wield it safely, for I have rarely experienced it,
somewhat to my relief! (In the next chapter I shall
comment on the public use of the 'gift of knowledge'
by a leader when ministering to an entire group.)
4. Counsellors, and a quiet place for counselling,

155

ought to be available at public healing services, not as advertised ministry, but as a private back-up ministry should pastoral situations arise. The distraught and very troubled can be gently led off to a quiet room where they can be in private and in caring hands.

5. Ministers involved with the Laying-on-of-hands need, on some occasions, to be quite firm if they have an individual who seems intent on pouring out his or her life history! Waiting, in hope, for a break is to court disaster! You must interrupt, and take this sort of line:

'I realize you have a lot you would like to share with me. But it is for the touch of Jesus Christ on your life that you have come. He knows *everything* about you and your situation. I'm going to ask him to touch your life and will express this by the Laying-on-of-hands – *now* – after a moment's quiet! If, after the service, you would like to talk with someone, approach one of the stewards and they will arrange it. Let's be quiet now for a moment or two, and then I will pray . . .'

Praying

I have already given various set forms (see above, chapter 6). If praying in response to someone's articulated need then note the following:

1. Do not be afraid to respond *formally* if a known formal prayer obviously applies. The more you know by heart the better.

2. Do not regard praying extempore or praying formally as rigid alternatives. A modification of something known may have both the strength of content and the merit of relevance.

3. If praying extempore, pray as you *can*, do not

pray as you can't! Do not pretend to be some spiritual giant, you are not out to impress anybody!

4. *Don't forget GOD*! A focus upon God, Father, Son and Holy Spirit will often eclipse and bypass problems of 'correct' words and prayers. If – as is likely for many of us most of the time! – you have no idea what God is doing or intends to do, base your prayer not on guesswork, but on what you know to be true. If there is a cripple before you, and, like most of us, you have no conviction whatever that he is going to leap up and run around the church, do not verbalize what you do not believe, but what you do.

God is the only person that we can speak about with utter confidence; his presence with us, his love for us, his faithfulness to us, his understanding of us. If in doubt, base your prayer on what you know about God rather than on guesswork at what he is doing or its future results.

5. In not forgetting God we will avoid the error of praying Godward prayers of diagnosis, in which all the sufferer's complaints are described to God for the second time in three minutes! In laying on hands we are ministering God's blessing manward, not underlining man's complaints Godward!

6. My own rule for most informal occasions in praying is, 'When in doubt, be *Trinitarian*'. When our ears and minds are awash with pastoral details a retreat into God and a God-based prayer is usually the solution (see my prayer on p. 81). The needy are not helped by thin religious sentiment, they need prayers of *strength*. This strength is not best achieved by volume, fervour or outlandish promises! The strength required is that of God himself. Trinitarian praying, focusing the character and work of the

Father, the Son and the Holy Spirit, provides strength of the right sort.

7. There is a price that we sometimes have to pay for such ministry, but it is very small when compared to the blessing God may give at our hands. Sometimes it really does 'take it out of you'.

Very early in my ordained ministry I was called in an emergency to anoint a child in hospital. Next day I kept stretching myself and moaning to my wife, 'I feel as if I've been heaving furniture!' Only when I was more experienced did I link the two. The best thing is simply to ignore any aches and pains, and never ever to put any significance on them either good or bad, but turn them into thanksgiving that probably something really was happening!

8. In general use the person's *name*. I would usually ask a person's name last thing before praying over them, and then immediately incorporate it into the prayer, whether formal or informal. (Asking it last has the added advantage of not having to ask twice because you have already forgotten! If you do forget, then the 'brother/sister' of Christian fellowship can be usefully employed!)

9. Perhaps the most important thing to learn in such ministry is to *let go*. As you move from person to person *leave* the last, not temporarily but for good (unless they reappear in later pastoral care). There is a great temptation to cling, and mentally and spiritually to 'mother' everything that comes our way. There are many causes for this. Among them are our own need to matter; our inability to be still; our pride in 'lording' it over others; our enjoyment of power; our desire to justify ourselves by our pastoral busyness, and so on.

Our Lord's command to Mary Magdalene not to cling to him (John 20:17) says much about the style of Christ's ministry, as well as about Mary! Earlier he had instructed the Apostles and the seventy to cope with rejection by a symbolic act of shaking the dust off their feet (Mark 6:11, Luke 10:10–11).

In ministering, our compassion will lead us to 'suffer with' those in pain, sorrow, and heartache. Our ministry will survive only if we learn to let go.

Use anything that works for you to accomplish this: a long walk, a hot bath and/or an Agatha Christie! Never carry today's pastoral load overnight for tomorrow. Drop it. Place it back in Father's hands where it belongs – and where it is safest! If God calls us to carry some load tomorrow he will give it afresh.

Do not be misled by nagging thoughts about not really caring and treating people casually. It is better to minister for four decades having learnt the discipline of letting go, than to minister for just four weeks because of a failure to do so!

Later disciples inherited Jesus's advice and took it: 'They stirred up persecution against Paul and Barnabas . . . So they shook the dust from their feet in protest against them and went to Iconium. And the disciples were filled with joy and with the Holy Spirit' (Acts 13:50–1). They had learned to let go, and their 'filling' of joy and the Holy Spirit probably required an earlier emptying of pastoral burdens. A good cook frequently washes her hands to prevent mix and muddle. We too need to start afresh.

Since we take neither the credit nor the blame for what does or does not happen it is inappropriate for the majority of us to keep records of such ministry or tabs on those involved. The reason there are few healing stories in this book is that I have very promptly let go of pastoral situations once I have ministered to them, and have hardly any recollections of any 'results'. This detachment has the added advantage that we come to each pastoral situation afresh, and are unlikely to fall into the trap of repeating yesterday's actions as a formula for today's success.

Once the art of touching has been learned, then comes the all-important art of letting go!

I entitled this chapter *Loving* because the actions that I have analysed and dissected are just love in action! It cannot be gleaned from a textbook, nor should one ever dictate our behaviour. In this next chapter I shall deal with a few important things that may be encountered and of which we need to have some understanding, including the falling phenomenon, exorcism, and the public exercise of the 'Word of Knowledge'.

What I have shared here will not equip you to minister, but it may give you, if called, the necessary confidence to touch others more appropriately in the Name of Christ.

1. Lancelot Sheppard's *The Curé d'Ars*, Burns and Oates, p. 89.

13

Encountering

There are certain things which we may encounter at a public healing service and it is useful to have some understanding of them.

The Falling Phenomenon

When a person is prayed over for healing they can gently collapse! The phenomenon accompanies certain ministers. In some circles it is assumed to have great spiritual significance and is called 'resting in the Spirit' or being 'slain by the Spirit'. Cardinal Suenens in his book *Resting in the Spirit* summarizes my thinking:

> An Anglican minister, J Richards, suggests that to begin with, we should adopt a neutral term that remains purely descriptive and does not make its spiritual content and interpretation a foregone conclusion . . . I endorse his suggestion. In short, I shall more frequently speak of 'falling' than 'resting' (pp. 17–18).

The phenomenon can occur with Spiritualists and others. It is not necessarily Christian or of the Holy Spirit. It is only Christian and of spiritual significance if it has *Christian results*. There is no means of knowing until afterwards!

Unfortunately some Christians have gone overboard on this, and the women attend meetings in slacks not skirts and 'catchers' are lined up deliberately! It is easy to see how such a gathering can create the phenomenon by its own mental expectancy!

We must avoid either maximizing it or minimizing it. It is best when the phenomenon is not expected or encouraged, then, if it takes place, it is more likely to be authentic. It has only twice accompanied my praying over people: both were unexpected – at least to me! The Communion rail is not the best place for it, although folk collapse in a very relaxed way and no one ever seems to hurt themselves! Ideally the person should be seated in a chair where they can gently 'rest in the Spirit' without keeling over.

If it happens do not worry about it. The person may be in a semi-conscious state for quite a time. In the context of a healing service it is likely that a deep healing is taking place. Many lives have been utterly transformed when God ministers in this way.

Falling has accompanied the lives of Christians as diverse as John Wesley and St Teresa of Avila. It diminished during Wesley's ministry and St Teresa recognized that the phenomenon could be caused by human weakness, feminine silliness or sheer exhibitionism! She advised the heads of religious Orders who had members prone to such manifestations to make them do plenty of hard work and not to let them spend over-long at their prayers![1] She clearly did not get too intense about it, and her attitude is a good one for us to share!

The phenomenon seems to accompany certain ministers, but most often they allow an expectancy to build up around it. It is neither a sign of special ministry nor of special blessing. Indeed it seems to happen more to the immature who are resisting God than to those who are most open to him.

There is no precise Scriptural equivalent, and the relevant material is dealt with in my booklet '*Resting in the Spirit*'. Suffice it to mention here that there is a difference between a *forward* falling in worship, and falling *backwards*. St Paul's well-known falling on the Damascus Road (Acts 9:4ff, 26:14) is sometimes taken as a precedent, but it did *not* result in him rising up healed and Spirit-filled, but blinded and in need of Ananias's ministry.

The main Scriptures are:

(a) 2 Chron. 5:14, the *priests* cannot stand in God's presence.

(b) Ezek. 1:28, *Ezekiel* falls face down in God's presence.

(c) Dan. 10:9, *Daniel* falls face down in his vision.

(d) Matt. 17:6, the *disciples* fall face down at the Transfiguration.

(e) Rev. 1:17, *John* falls at the feet of the Son of Man.

(f) Mark 9:14–27, the *epileptic demoniac* collapses during ministry.

(g) John 18:6, the *crowd* fall down backwards at Jesus's arrest.

(h) Acts 9:4, 26:14, *Saul and companions* fall on the Damascus Road.

Most falling is forward and a response to the presence of God. Some falling is a clash between good and evil, as (f), (g) and possibly (h) above.

If you have not yet encountered this phenomenon you probably will. It erupts in many different traditions. The Salvation Army call it 'having a glory fit!', and Cardinal Suenens notes with some unease that at a service at Lourdes 'priests in vestments were seen falling like ninepins'!

When praying over others many will be anxious that they might find themselves ministering to someone whose malady is beyond their experience or understanding.

'What am I to do if someone comes up for the Laying-on-of-hands and says "I'm possessed"?'

This is where the spiritual preparation for the service (see pp. 113–14) is highly relevant. If, through our prayers, God has drawn together a gathering of his choice, prepared those of his choice for the event, and kept away those who would not be helped, then it may be assumed that the spiritual and personal resources at such a gathering will be carefully chosen to accomplish God's healing work.

So relax! Do not be panicked by a claim to being possessed. No truly 'possessed' person is voluntarily going to attend a healing service and ask for the Laying-on-of-hands! Very much milder forms of oppression or overshadowing of some sort can be ministered to on such occasions simply by the Lord's Prayer – which is, in itself, a prayer for deliverance.

The church's authority over evil can be exercised (no, that's not a misprint!) by a word of *restraint* or 'binding', not only by casting out. In the unlikely event of there being any sort of disturbance, then an authoritative 'In the Name of Jesus Christ be quiet!' will subdue any evil forces operating within the person – while not, of course, restricting their personal freedom to kick up a fuss if they wish! (The Church only binds *evil*, never people – that is the job of the devil!)

Do not over-react or act over-hastily. Do not hesitate to summon a senior minister if you feel unsure. If you are ministering in pairs, then any unexpected happening is not encountered alone, but with the support of another.

Time and time again I have witnessed the Lord directing those in need to those who spiritually and humanly are best able to help them.

For further reading see my introductory *The Minister and the Deliverance Ministry*, and *Exorcism, Deliverance and Healing*, or for a fuller treatment my *But Deliver Us From Evil*.

Group Ministering without Laying on Hands

Most of what I have written assumes that the Laying-on-of-hands will be given at a public healing service. In most cases it is so, but not always.

When, for the Fountain Trust, Sr Briege McKenna (author of *Miracles Do Happen*) led a service of healing in a packed Central Hall Westminster, she simply taught and then prayed for those present. She prayed for those with physical needs, emotional needs, those with broken relationships, the bereaved, and so on.

This is rarer, but must not be thought odd. It was primarily by the *word* that Jesus healed (see above p. 76). Of the individual healings recorded, very nearly half make no record of any touching, and of these cases less than half were demoniacs. Christ healed three folk at a distance, all children: the Syro-Phoenician girl (Mark 7:29–30), the official's son (John 4:50–3), and the centurion's slave (Luke 7:6–10), – who Matthew, in the Greek, noted was a 'boy' (8:6).

Prayers for healing without laying on hands occur during most times of intercession for the sick at regular worship, some of whom will be present and others not.

There are occasions when worship – with no 'healing' label or intent – has been the occasion of great personal transformations and healings. I believe that it is of the essence of worship to change and heal, and that worship should be the offering of the whole person and the blessing of the whole person. Good worship is healing. It is not worship that needs changing in order for it to become healing, but for the worshippers to re-evaluate worship and enjoy its healing dimensions.

'Word of Knowledge' Ministries

There are some charismatic ministers who exercise what is often called the 'Word of Knowledge' (see above pp. 154–5) not in one-to-one ministry but in relation to an entire congregation.

A typical example would be to say that the Lord has made them aware of someone present with e.g. asthma whom he wishes to heal. The speaker might then try to identify the individual concerned, or might simply pray for them before being made aware of another person's needs. When I have witnessed such ministry it has always been discreet in terms of personal details.

Many would testify to the Lord healing them on such occasions.

From my limited observation and experiences of this I would say that there are some very fine and wonderful examples of this ministry and many that trouble me, and that I am not alone in these two reactions. My concern is when the individual(s) is not precisely specified. Every person present with the same or similar symptoms wonders whether it applies to them. In a congregation I have sat amidst very considerable confusion and anxiety.

Nudge, nudge, 'Doesn't he mean *you* dear?'

'Oh, I don't think . . . er . . . isn't it her over there?'

'No, silly, you were only telling me this morning how much your head was aching . . .'

'Ought I to stand up . . .?'

'Too late, luv, he's off onto something else now! I'm sure he meant you, though!'

'Oh dear, what should I do . . .?'

'Shhh! Be quiet!'

I do not question the ability of the minister to hear what God is saying. That would be presumptive on my part. I do not doubt the Lord's use of such ministry to bring healing.

My unease rests on two things.

The first is the exercise of spiritual gifts in a way which is assumed to be of the Lord and which leaves no room whatever for other Christian leaders to weigh or discern it. I think this is a spiritually dangerous exercise that is very likely to fuel power-hungry individualists.

My second reason for unease is my conviction that it is a characteristic of the devil to spread confusion, but of the Holy Spirit to bring order. If the exercise of a gift of the Holy Spirit brings confusion, I am left with only two possible conclusions: either it is not of the Holy Spirit, or it is ministered wrongly.

In large gatherings it *is* possible for individual insights to be 'weighed' by other leaders.

I remember being in the sanctuary with about twenty others at a Mass in Westminster Cathedral. We were gathered to 'filter' contributions of words, prophecies, etc., that members of the congregation wished to offer. What was accepted was good and was offered for the building up of the Body of Christ. The vague, anaemic, and unScriptural offerings we rejected. Each offering was written down and passed among the group of us for our thumbs up or down! It was a little ponderous, perhaps the numbers were too great, but I greatly approved it in principle. There was no confusion and what was shared had the authority of the Church behind it.

I would like to see this particular style of ministry operating on the Biblical two-by-two basis, i.e. done as a pair with the checking and enriching of the second person. Perhaps one would discern God's general word while the other might be gifted to focus it and thus avoid its usual ambiguity and confusion.

This would at least place it nearer Scripture. It may be a legitimate development from Scripture, but it seems to me that there are no Biblical precedents for it and little Biblical encouragement.

1. St Teresa of Avila, *Interior Castle*, VI, §2, etc.

14

Inspiring

There are countless impressive healing stories in the relevant literature that I might borrow to conclude this book. My choice for inspiration is not strictly speaking even a 'healing' story. It is not extraordinary, indeed it is its basic *ordinariness* that I find so overwhelming and encouraging. That ordinary folk like you and me may be called to enter into such things is just beyond words. If you can 'catch' what it is saying then you will have touched the heart of this book.

A young child was taken by his mother to a service of Holy Communion. After his mother had received the bread and wine, the minister prayed for the child with the Laying-on-of-hands. (Such a blessing was usual for those who were not confirmed – the child was not ill.)

When he had returned with his mother to their seats, he leant over and whispered to her, 'Mummy, what is the name of that nice man who *poured that lovely warm oil all over me?*'

Thy blessed unction from above
Is comfort, life and fire of love;
Enable with perpetual light
The dullness of our blinded sight.

Bibliographies

Authoritative Documents

Archbishops' Commission Report 1958, *The Church's Healing Ministry*, abridged John Richards, Marshall-Pickering/Renewal Servicing, 1986.

Booth, Howard, *Healing is Wholeness*, Methodist Church Division of Social Responsibility/Churches' Council for Health and Healing, 1987.

Division of Social Responsibility, *Services of Healing*, Methodist Church (undated).

Health and Healing Group, *Health and Healing in the Bible*, Stanley Thomas *et al*, Department of Mission, Baptist Union, 1979.

Health and Healing Group, *Services of Healing*, Baptist Union, 1983.

McManus, Fr Jim, C ss R, *The Healing Power of the Sacraments*, Redemptorist Publications, Alton, 1984.

Ministry of Healing Committee, *Health and Healing: a Study Kit*, United Reformed Church, 1982.

Details of principal publications mentioned in text

*Denotes of particular importance

Administration of Holy Unction and the Laying on of Hands, SPCK 1935.

But Deliver Us From Evil, John Richards, Darton, Longman and Todd 1974.

Children and the Healing Ministry (pamphlet), John Richards, Renewal Servicing 1986.

170

Chrism (quarterly), Editor: Penelope Turing, Guild of St Raphael, St Marylebone Parish Church.

Christian Healing, Dr Evelyn Frost, Mowbray 1940.

Christian Healing Ministry, Bishop Morris Maddocks, SPCK 1981.

*The Church's Healing Ministry (Commission Report 1958), abridged John Richards, Marshall-Pickering and Renewal Servicing 1986.

The Church's Ministry of Healing (Commission Report), Church Information Office 1958, (out of print).

Exorcism, Deliverance and Healing, John Richards, Grove Books, Nottingham 1976.

Faith and Healing (pamphlet), John Richards, Renewal Servicing 1984.

From the Pinnacle of the Temple: Faith or Presumption? Charles Farah, Jr, Logos International (undated).

Gospel and Medicine (pamphlet), John Richards, Renewal Servicing 1985.

Healing and Christianity: In Ancient Thought and Modern Times, Morton T. Kelsey, SCM 1973.

Healing Is Wholeness, Howard Booth, Methodist Church Division of Social Responsibility/Churches' Council for Health and Healing 1987.

Healing Miracles, Dr Rex Gardner, Darton, Longman and Todd 1986.

The Healing Power of the Sacraments, Fr J. McManus, Redemptorist Publications, Alton 1984.

Healing Services, United Reformed Church 1982.

*Health and Healing: Studies in NT Principles and Practice, Dr John Wilkinson, Handsel Press, Edinburgh 1980.

Health and Healing: Study Kit, United Reformed Church 1982.

Heart of Healing, Revd George Bennett, Arthur James 1971.

Laying on of Hands (pamphlet), John Richards, Renewal Servicing 1982.

The Lord is Our Healer, Canon John Gunstone, Hodder and Stoughton 1986.

The Minister and the Deliverance Ministry, John Richards, Renewal Servicing 1983.

'The Ministry of Healing' in *Convictions*, Lord Coggan, Hodder and Stoughton 1975.

Miracle at Crowhurst, Revd George Bennett, Arthur James 1970.

Miracles Do Happen, Sr Briege McKenna osc, Veritas Publications 1988.

*Prayers for Healing, Canon John Gunstone, Highland Books 1987.

The Person of Christ and the Power of Healing (tape), Bishop Michael Marshall, Guild of St Raphael 1987.

Power Evangelism, John Wimber, Hodder and Stoughton 1985.

Power Healing, John Wimber, Hodder and Stoughton 1986.

The Power to Heal, Francis MacNutt, Ave Maria Press 1977.

Renewal In Worship, Bishop Michael Marshall, Marshalls 1982.

Resting in the Spirit: A Controversial Phenomenon, L-J. Cardinal Suenens, Veritas, Dublin 1987.

'*Resting in the Spirit*', John Richards, Renewal Servicing 1983.

Services of Healing, Baptist Union 1983.

Services of Healing, Methodist Church (undated).

Some Thoughts on Faith Healing, V. Edmunds and C. G. Scorer, Christian Medical Fellowship and Tyndale Press 1956.

To Heal As Jesus Healed, Barbara Shlemon, Ave Maria Press.

Twenty-Four Healing Prayers (pamphlet), John Richards, Renewal Servicing 1985.

Understanding Anointing (pamphlet), John Richards, Renewal Servicing 1981.

Way of Life (quarterly), Editor: James Breese, Guild of Health, 26 Queen Anne St, London.

We Believe in Healing, ed. Dr Ann England, Highland Books, Crowborough 1986.

Your Very Good Health: Directory of Groups involved in Health and Healing in Britain, Churches' Council for Health and Healing 1980.

Books, etc. not mentioned in the text.

Baker, John P., *Salvation and Wholeness*, Fountain Trust 1973.

Benedictine Monk, A, *The Ministry of Healing Prayer*, National Service Committee for Catholic Charismatic Renewal 1984.

Booth, Howard, *Healing Experiences*, Bible Reading Fellowship 1985.

—*In Search of Health and Wholeness*, Methodist Church, Division of Social Responsibility 1985.

Buchanan, Colin and David Wheaton, *Liturgy for the Sick*, Grove Books, Nottingham 1983.

Botting, Michael, *Pastoral and Liturgical Ministry to the Sick*, Grove Books 1978.

Dale, David H., *The Bible and Healing*, United Reformed Church 1983.

Faricy, Robert, *Praying for Inner Healing*, SCM 1979.

Gibbs, Eddie, 'John Wimber – A friend who causes me to wonder', *Renewal*, no. 123, June, 1986.

Glennon, Canon Jim, *How Can I Find Healing?* Hodder and Stoughton 1984.

—*Your Healing Is Within You*, Hodder and Stoughton 1978.

Goldingay, John, 'Theology and Healing', *Churchman*, vol. 92, no. 1, 1978.

Gregg, David, *Ministry to the Sick: An Introduction*, Grove Books 1978.

Gusmer, Prof. Charles W., *The Ministry of Healing in the Church of England*, Alcuin Club/Mayhew-McCrimmon, Great Wakering 1974.

Hamel Cooke, Christopher, *Health Is For God*, Arthur James 1986.

Harrison, Alan, *Preparation for the Church's Ministry of Healing*, Guild of Health (undated).

Howell, David, *Healing and Wholeness in the N.T.*, DHM, Crowhurst.

Hutchison, Harry, *Healing Through Worship*, Eyre and Spottiswoode 1981.

MacNutt, Francis, *Healing*, Ave Maria Press 1974.

Methuen, Rev John, 'Healing Service', *Chrism*, vol. XXI, no. 8, 1978.

Ministry to the Sick (Authorized Alternative Services), Central Board of Finance, Church of England 1983.

Moss, Dr Kay, 'Healing Services', *Way of Life*, vol. 20, no. 1, 1988.

O'Connor, Fr Edward, csc, *The Laying on of Hands*, Dove Publications, USA 1969.

Piller, Bishop Kenneth (Chairman of Working Party), *Guidelines for Healing Services*, St Alban's Diocese 1983.

Rahner, Karl, sj, *The Anointing of the Sick*, Dimension Books, USA 1970.

Richards, John (and see p. 175), 'A Total Gospel for Total Man', *Christian Herald*, 114/48, 1980.

—*Getting Healing Under Way*, Renewal Servicing 1981.

—'Gifts of Healings', *Colomen*, Renewal in Wales, no. 7, 1984.

—'Healing Foundations', *Renewal*, no. 135, 1987.

—'Laying on of Hands and Healing', *Chrism*, Vol. XXV, no. 2, 1985.

—'Out to Heal', *Theological Renewal*, no. 13, 1979.

—'Sacramental and Charismatic Contributions to Healing', *Chrism*, vol. XXIV, no. 4, 1982.

—'What About Public Healing Services?' *Chrism*, vol. XXIV, no. 7, 1983.

'Service of Healing', *Chrism*, vol. XXIV, no. 12, 1984.

Service of Healing, St Marylebone Parish Church, London.

Smail, Tom, 'The Healing Church', *Renewal*, no. 115, 1985.

'Spotlight on Validation', *Health and Healing*, no. 8, 1985.

Turnbull, James, 'Further Thoughts on Healing Services', *Way of Life*, vol. 15, no. 2, 1983.

—'Pastoral Care of Those attending Healing Services', *Way of Life*, vol. 15, no. 3, 1983.

—'Some Thoughts on Healing Services', *Way of Life*, vol. 15, no. 1, 1983.

Wylie, Revd. George, *The Place and Purpose of Services of Healing*, Divine Healing Mission, Crowhurst.

Other relevant publications of John Richards

Among the pamphlets available from Renewal Servicing, P.O. Box 17, Shepperton, Middx. TW17 8NU, are:

Children and The Healing Ministry
Faith & Healing
Gospel and Medicine
Healers, Gifts and Healing
Laying on of Hands
Notes for Healing Services
The Problem of Fear
Questions and Answers – Resting in the Spirit
Suffering and Gospel
Tears – Gift of the Spirit?
The Ordinary Christian and Spiritual Warfare
Twenty-Four Healing Prayers
Understanding Anointing
Why Am I Not Healed?
Wilderness – The Christian Experience

These, and another fifteen pamphlet titles, are available from the address above, cost by post (UK) 1–30p, 2–50p, 5–£1.

Organizations

Mentioned in the text

(This excludes the list on pp. 18–19.)

Churches' Council for Health and Healing, St Marylebone Parish Church, Marylebone Rd, NW1 5LT

Divine Healing Mission, The Old Rectory, Crowhurst, Battle, Sussex, TN33 9AD

Guild of Health, Edward Wilson House, 26 Queen Anne St, W1M 9LB

Guild of St Raphael, St Marylebone Parish Church, Marylebone Rd, NW1 5LT

Not mentioned in the text

See the Directory *Your Very Good Health*, published by the Churches' Council for Health and Healing.

Biblical Index

178

Index of Main Topics

The numerals refer to the chapter